JOURNEYS, KITTENS
AND CASTLES . . . OLD BOYFRIENDS,
BEES, AND WHALES!

- Do you dream about specific kinds of food, such as chocolate or fruit?
- Do you dream about misplacing your baby?
- Are cats frequent visitors in your dreams?
- Do stars like Brad Pitt or Leonardo DiCaprio appear in your dreams?
- Do you dream about flowers? Are they in perfect bloom or do they need water?
- Are certain colors, such as blue or red, dominant in your dreams?
- Do you dream you're swimming with dolphins?

Discover the fascinating and special meanings these dream symbols and images have for mothers- (and fathers-) to-be. Begin the journey to the frontiers of your unconscious mind to achieve intimate, personal contact with your baby's soul and personality. And bring harmony and a wondrous awareness to your pregnancy and beyond with . . .

THE MOTHER-TO-BE'S DREAM BOOK

THE MOTHER-TO-BE'S DREAM BOOK

Understanding the Dreams of Pregnancy

Raïna M. Paris

WARNER BOOKS

A Time Warner Company

Copyright © 2000 by Raïna Paris and Andrew Ridgeway
All rights reserved.

Warner Books, Inc., 1271 Avenue of the Americas, New York, NY 10020
Visit our Web site at www.twbookmark.com

 A Time Warner Company

Printed in the United States of America
First Printing: April 2000
10 9 8 7 6 5 4 3 2 1

Library of Congress Cataloging-in-Publication Data

Paris, Raïna.
    The mother-to-be's dream book : understanding the dreams of pregnancy / Raïna Paris.
        p. cm.
    ISBN 0-446-67524-5 (trade pbk.)
    1. Women's dreams. 2. Dream interpretation. 3. Pregnancy—Psychological aspects.   I. Title.
BF1099.W65 P37 2000
154.6'32—dc21

                                                                    99-049032
                                                                    CIP

Book design and text composition by L&G McRee
Cover design by Carolyn Lechter
Cover illustration by Jenny Tilden-Wright

To my godson Talon Nathaniel Hadfield

CONTENTS

CONTENTS

Contents

CONTENTS

Contents

PROLOGUE

I have found a way to combine two of my life's passions in *The Mother-to-Be's Dream Book*, and for that I am very grateful. The first passion began when I was seven years old. I remember being in the middle of a luscious dream when the alarm clock rudely interrupted me. I was so incensed at being torn away from the blissful experience of riding bareback on a wild horse who had adopted me into his family that I decided to go right back to sleep with the hopes of reentering my delightful dream.

I summoned the feelings of the dream and its powerful imagery to guide me back into the story and promptly fell back asleep, picking up right where I had left off. During the dream I was both thrilled and aware that I had accomplished my goal. I was amazed by my abilities. I was a determined little girl.

This event stirred in me a long passion for the realm of dreams and fairy tales. As an adult I began studying the unconscious and practicing spiritual work. This led me back to dream analysis. I realized that it was an essential component of the soul's ability to communicate and participate in the creation and transformation of man and woman. From the beginning, my dreams have been a guiding force in my own life. They gave me hope and showed me a way at a time when I thought there was none. They reconnected me with my ancestors. They helped me figure out what I needed to look at in analysis. And they showed me what myths I had been living by. For me, dreams have been a direct connection to my own soul, my most authentic self.

Dreams are like the signals of the soul emerging from our unconscious in the same way that symptoms can emerge from the body. They do not lie. In fact, dreams can show us what is happening in the body before it becomes pathology. Whatever light or shadow we carry is made clear through our dreams. They are our teachers. Dream analysis can be a very powerful journey to embark on. This is vibrantly apparent during the process of pregnancy, as you will learn through the course of this book.

My second passion has to do with motherhood itself. When I was twelve years old, I fell in love for the first time. He was a 2½-year-old little boy named David. With his dark curls, olive skin, and deep black eyes, he looked uncannily like me. It was during my summer vacation, on the north coast of France, in Normandy. I was an only child, and left to my own devices. David had been left to the care of two older women, who knitted away the day under a parasol. The baby was left to play alone in the sand with his small red pail.

To my vivid twelve-year-old mind, the two nannies were really old witches who were keeping the little prince prisoner. The first day I asked innocently if I could play with him, they agreed. Little did they know I was a heroine in disguise coming to rescue a toddler who looked as lonely as I felt. The love and trust that developed between us over the next few weeks was the most overwhelming feeling of unconditional love I had ever experienced. It was as if we had known each other forever. If I had known what reincarnation meant at that time, I would have believed we had been mother and child in a past life.

I totally surrendered my heart to him. A deep maternal bond was established, to the point that, without any coaching, he began to call me Mother. When the boy's mother overheard this one day, she promptly talked to my mother, and I was forbidden to ever see David again. The summer came to a close and I returned to school.

In the months and years that followed, the memory of this unconditional love between two children sustained me through many difficult moments in my adolescence—my parents' divorce, the deaths of family and friends. This bond of love between mother and child, I am convinced, transcends time and space. It is truly bigger than we are and teaches us to be better than we think we can be. This book about the dreams of mothers-to-be reflects my belief that such a bond is created and developed through our dream world before the child is even born.

This practical book includes information and exercises to help you (and your mate) bond with your unborn child. It follows the development of the child over the three trimesters and will help you to understand your dreams during each stage of your pregnancy. You will notice that as your baby develops your dreams will change—as will you. By analyzing and understanding your dreams you will learn about your anxieties, fears, and thoughts about your baby. I have also included personal accounts of dreams of women—and some men—that I hope will enrich your own pregnancy and your relationship with your child, and help strengthen the lifelong bond between the two of you.

ACKNOWLEDGMENTS

I am grateful beyond the measure of these words to my agent Laura Dail and editor Diana Baroni who conspired to create this opportunity for me to put together my passion for dreams and my passion for the bond between mother and child in *The Mother-to-Be's Dream Book*.

This book could not have been written without the loving support of my dear friends Odette and Merrill, the spiritual steadiness of Reverend Carol Traylor, and the insightful comments of Andrei Ridgeway who helped me curb my natural European tendency to write what most American-born literati dismiss as run-on sentences (like this one).

Last, but most important, I want to thank all the women who have made this book possible. Their stories are the heart, the spine, and the liver of this book: Sybil,

ACKNOWLEDGMENTS

Hope, Juliette, Lynette, Kari, Tracy, Jenny, Dayna, Deedee, Nancy, Alexis, Lynda, Marie, Maddix, Lisa, Lucy, Susan, Mina, and many more whose names have been changed to preserve the privacy they craved, especially after the birth of their newborn baby.

I also want to give thanks to the fathers, John, Spencer, Walter, Reverend Nirvana Reginald Gayle, and all the others who chose to remain anonymous, yet made such a beautiful contribution to this book.

And finally, I feel so grateful to have been part of such a breathtaking adventure. My heart is filled with blessings for all the beautiful children who have been born since this book was first started and without whom none of this would have been written.

Thank you.

The Nature of Dreams

"Man is a genius when he is dreaming."

—*Akira Kurosawa*

The exhilaration and sheer joy of finding out that you are pregnant can be overwhelming. So congratulations are definitely in order. And yet, like dreaming, pregnancy is, for most women, an essential and normal part of our life cycle. In the state of heightened awareness that pregnancy provides, the dreaming cycle itself can become an invaluable asset for a mother-to-be, like clues to a newly discovered treasure map. Through our dreams we can learn about ourselves and our unborn children.

In our waking state, we use a limited part of our brain, but during sleep we are open to multidimensional realms that can embrace all times, past and future.

While we dream, we rest and renew ourselves, and even heal. Our unconscious is free to deal with things that we are unable to acknowledge during waking hours. We fly, we change our physical form, we swim with dolphins and run with wolves. In our dreams we come face-to-face with all of our fears, our desires, and our most personal demons.

In ancient times, the dreaming mind was thought to be connected to the divine. From Plato to the prophets in the Bible, dreams were considered messages from the gods. In Native American traditions, young warriors would let their dreams lead them on a vision quest, helping them to align with the forces of Nature and their higher self.

It is only in recent times that dreams have lost their capacity to guide us. Freudian psychology might be partially responsible for this, by narrowing everything down to a sexual interpretation. And the materialistic realism of our scientific society may also be responsible as it has closed our minds to the greater potential of dreaming.

It is no accident, however, that in a therapeutic context the analysis of dreams is still considered an extraordinary gateway for self-discovery and self-knowledge. Dreaming is the way the soul communicates with our conscious self. Through symbols and pictures, it creates meaningful stories in a language uniquely personal to the dreamer.

Some dreams come to us in the form of guidance, pulling us out of sleep with a sudden realization that changes our lives. Other dreams speak through unique characters, who have a seemingly endless flow of imagination. There are also dreams that predict the future, giving us the details of an event that has yet to occur so that we may be better prepared. There are worry dreams and anxiety dreams, and dreams that reveal our deepest desires. Some dreams can even resolve psychological conflicts, like a master therapist, bringing our psyche into better harmony.

What you will discover in this book is that dreams that occur during pregnancy are full of such revelations about you and your child. Thanks to the dreams of all the women interviewed, I was able to discover a dream pattern that loosely follows that of the first, second, and third trimesters. These women's dreams, and the exercises provided at the end of each chapter will help you reach a deeper understanding of your own dreams. You will be able to discern your own dream patterns as your child grows within you.

The second part of the book centers around premonitions and other psychic aspects of pregnancy dreams. The research in this area is so plentiful and interesting, it cannot be ignored. I have also included a section on dreams of the fathers. Fathers-to-be are as involved in the pregnancy process as you are. Some of the fathers' dreams were full of signposts and predictions. When addressed in a conscious manner, they can help ease the tension between the couple that often arises at this time, whether because of financial concerns or just about bringing a new being into the world.

The last two sections of the book are more specifically geared toward the art of dreaming itself. They bring into focus the images and symbols that more often recur in dreams during pregnancy. Finally, I have included a series of exercises to help you increase your ability to remember and understand your own dreams.

Though they often appear like riddles, always remember that these dreams are the language of your own soul, your most intimate and authentic self.

Your dreams can be a gateway to forgiveness, understanding, and growth. They are the meeting place between spirit and matter. They can bring new perspective to your daily life, a fuller circle of existence that is not bound by this earthly body, and touch the frontiers of your soul. They can bring you more personal and intimate contact with your baby's soul and personality long before he/she is ever born.

PART I

❦

The Evolution
of Dreams during
Pregnancy

❦

"I am gathering the riches from my dreaming travels so that I may remember more of myself than I knew before."

—*The Transitional Dreamer*

A woman's dreaming life deepens the moment she decides to become pregnant. It is as if the soul and the body of the woman conspire together to create space for the future baby. This space is as much a psychic space as a physical one. It is an opening in the woman's consciousness, a link between the physical and spiritual worlds, where healing can occur and the mystery of life is a living reality.

A pregnant woman's dreams are a rich tapestry where old lovers appear and animals become wise guardians, taking the woman on a journey in which she becomes the living embodiment of Nature's creation. A pregnant woman can meet her unborn child through her dreams, understand the language of the heart by swimming with dolphins and facing her own childhood fears. Such dreams are a lifeline available to a woman on this unfathomable journey. Pregnancy dreams are Nature's way of assisting the woman through the process of transformation from woman to mother. It is a soul-enriching experience, and whatever information a woman receives in her sleep is an invaluable gift.

This part of the book thoroughly examines the types of dreams specific to pregnancy, as well as their evolution through the first, second, and third trimester, providing a guide for expectant mothers.

CHAPTER ONE

Conception and the First Trimester: Dreams of the Past

Around the time of conception and well into the first trimester, a woman's dreams will act as a therapeutic tool to help her clear up unresolved issues from the past, so that she may be psychologically prepared for her new offspring. Dreams of the past often appear at this time, including images of old homes and family members or friends with whom relationships need to be worked out—a father, a mother, ex-boyfriends, for instance. These dreams, though not directly related to the pregnancy, are the way the unconscious brings to the surface certain issues that might interfere with the mother-to-be's capacity to mother her child. For instance, many dreams have to do with the mother-to-be's own childhood. The dreams will help her look at her relationship to her mother and father, and how the beliefs and patterns she established early on in her life affect her current ideas about mothering and babyhood. It is an opportunity for the mother-to-be to examine, challenge, and question these beliefs and old patterns, some of which are no longer useful.

Dreams of lost love also appear at this time. They help the mother-to-be to look at her old patterns and let go of unfinished business with ex-lovers. These dreams are also a way for the unconscious to help the mother-to-be say good-bye to her days as a maiden.

These early dreaming cycles have a sense of urgency about them. They help a woman eliminate the restrictive patterns in her life that might prevent her from flourishing as a mother. They are Nature's way of making the baby feel welcome. The mother-to-be usually experiences daily life with an increase in self-awareness. Early pregnancy dreams lead a woman to wholeness, drawing up broken pieces from the past and forming them into a new, revitalized human being. These dreams provide an honest mirror to look into for the courageous and the willing, and the best kind of therapeutic help, the one only your own soul can give you. Let's discuss these types of dreams and look at some examples.

Dreams of Childhood

Having a baby is a mental idea before it becomes a physical reality. In the idea phase, it is a powerful catalyst for change. It animates a woman's unconscious and helps her remember and recover parts of herself that she might have lost over time. Such was the case with a woman I interviewed. She had a dream in which she met herself at various ages. The dream characters she saw in her sleep were reflections of who she used to be, both as a teenager and a young woman. There was also something else about the dream that was interesting. She and her husband had recently agreed on a name for a girl, and the name appeared vividly in the dream. Not only was her unconscious bringing up aspects from the past, it was also showing her that she was on the right track, that her intuitive connection with the child was already established. Here is the dream of the past the woman experienced after she decided that she wanted to have a child—at this point she had not even conceived:

> *I am in the lobby at a theater with my husband and some other people, including what looks like a dozen schoolgirls, approximately thirteen years old. My husband and I are with Laura and her friend. Laura is younger than me, about twenty-six or twenty-seven. We look alike. Many people think we are sisters in real life. Everyone is beginning to go into the theater to watch the show. I lag behind and happen to notice an old leather eyeglass case lying on the ground. Engraved on its cover is the name of the child I have been thinking about in my waking life. I call out the name, brandishing the leather case like a prize above my head. The schoolgirl to whom the case belongs answers. She is tomboyish, with curly black hair. She looks like me as a young girl. She thanks me. Then I see that Laura, my young friend, has also misplaced some things. I retrieve her thick leather Day-Timer and her checkbook, which also con-*

tains her driver's license. I am very proud of
finding all these lost precious things. They didn't
even know they had lost them and here I am
finding them and returning them to their owners.
I wake up.

After observing the characters in her dream, the
woman came to realize that the thirteen-year-old and
the twenty-six-year-old looked like two younger ver-
sions of herself. She also discovered that these two
characters represented periods of her life in which she
felt very lost and alone. In the dream, the woman finds
articles that bring resolution to these challenging times.
She recovers for each character an object that symbolizes their ability to function in the world in a way that
she was not able to at those ages in her life. By naming
her desire to have a child, she has set into motion a
cycle of healing.

Another woman I interviewed had such disturbing
dreams during her first trimester (when her hormones
were at their most energetic level) that she sought out
the help of a therapist for the first time in her life. Her
own parental issues, especially with her father, had
broken through to her consciousness in such a strong
manner that she could not avoid them anymore. Her
work with the therapist helped tremendously. She
learned how to be present with the process of her own
pregnancy, not just physically, but mentally and spiritually as well. Occurring only days apart, here are the
dreams that convinced her to see a therapist:

First dream:

> I am alone with the new baby who is asleep in
> his room. I am naked. A burglar with a mask
> comes through the glass door. I am in my child-
> hood home. There is a feeling of great danger for
> me and the baby. I feel very vulnerable. I can't
> see who the burglar is. He is holding a big
> hammer. If I go to pick up my new baby, he will
> catch us. If I run to the next house to get help,
> I'll be leaving the baby alone with the burglar. I
> wake up in despair focusing on this difficult
> choice. I feel in my mind that I probably
> wouldn't leave the baby and we would get killed
> together.

Second dream:

> There is a weird family reunion outdoors. I am
> in a small hot tub with my baby. We are naked.
> The rest of my family is in another bigger pool.
> As I get out of the hot tub, three men arrive on
> bikes. They are very threatening and I feel very
> vulnerable, because I am naked holding my
> baby. I try to call my family but they don't hear
> me. Eventually my father comes over. He
> doesn't seem to realize these men are threatening
> my life and the life of my baby. Instead of pro-
> tecting me, he starts chatting with them. It is
> very upsetting to me that my father cannot see
> how dangerous the situation is for a naked
> woman with a baby. Eventually, the men go
> away. They lose interest in me and my child.
> Apparently my father did help out, but not in the
> way I wanted him to.

In both dreams, there are several elements commonly found in the dreams of pregnant women. First, there is a feeling of vulnerability, which is a standard emotion women feel in early pregnancy. Second, there is a recurring theme of nakedness. In both dreams, the woman is without clothing; she is bare and accessible to the threatening strangers. And third, the woman feels the need to protect her child. This instinct also becomes apparent in the early stages of pregnancy. The fact that the dreamer feels protective is a sign that her defense systems are in working order. She is being prepared for the arduous task of motherhood.

All of these above characteristics usually appear in the first trimester. What makes these dreams noteworthy is the context and setting in which they appear and, of course, the characters present. In both dreams there is a deadly, threatening intrusion. In the first dream, the woman is in her childhood home with a flimsy glass door between her and the outside world. Her only choice is no choice. *Staying with her baby in her childhood home means death for both of them.* In the second dream, the woman's family is nearby, but they do not respond. When her father finally comes to her aid, he misunderstands the situation. *He doesn't take care of her and the child but chats with the potential killers instead.*

By examining these dreams, it became excruciatingly clear to the woman that as a child she never felt supported by her family. Just as in the dreams, she felt completely vulnerable, exposed, with no one to help her. The feeling of desolation and alarm present in the dreams woke her up to the reality of her own childhood, forcing her to face the feelings she still carried inside her while pregnant. Driven by the desire to do what was best for her child and for herself, she chose to examine her past consciously in therapy.

This journey was for her a very different experience from that she had during her first pregnancy. The first time around she was a career woman who had never been interested in babies, and although she was excited, becoming a mother was something she knew very little about. She was mostly involved in the physical process, the changes in her body, cravings, and the like. However, when she became pregnant the second time, she knew on a deeper level what was involved in becoming a mother. She had already gone through the process of giving birth. She knew what it felt like to have a soul connection with another being. She was now prepared to deal with the psychic baggage that had been revealed to her through her pregnancy dreams. The more she uncovered in therapy, the clearer the connection to her unborn child became.

Dayna's dreams during her first trimester were also peppered with dreams from the past.

> *I am in a big old ocean liner. It's kind of run-down. Rustic but comfortable. I am with my family. There is a great celebration going on . . . a wedding. It lasts at least two days because I remember eating breakfast while the sun was coming up on the horizon. Somehow the sunrise lets me know that however fun and comfortable this trip is, it's time for me to go. I decide to escape. I'm not the only one; some strangers are also getting into the lifeboats. They are crowded. The only way for me to get into a lifeboat is to*

jump into the ocean itself and swim to a boat that
has room for me. I make it to a lifeboat and there
are only strangers on it, but I feel calm, confident
that I'm doing what I'm supposed to do, even if it
doesn't seem to make sense that I'm leaving the
comfort of my old family on the ship. The whole
atmosphere of the dream is fairy-tale–like and the
colors are very vivid. All the strangers seem to be
people my age. I wake up thinking that I'm preg-
nant, I'm really pregnant!

After we looked at the dream together it became
clear that Dayna was moving away from her familiar
life, symbolized by the old rustic ocean liner. In doing
this, she had to release the safety of her family in order
to step into her new existence. Although there was a
wedding going on (which is a great metaphor for the
creation of a baby), something changed for her with the
sunrise. She had suddenly become conscious that she
was taking in the food of a new life. At that crucial
moment of her "breaking the fast," eating breakfast, she
decided to get off the old boat. She was literally getting
into a whole new life by getting into a "lifeboat"
without her family. In the dream, before getting into
the lifeboat, she had to jump straight into the deep,
unbounded ocean. This is the way the dream deals with
what is happening in her body, a transformation as powerful and limitless as the ocean itself.

Some dreams of the past are not meant as a letting go
but more as a nourishing memory that provides comfort
for the soul of the pregnant woman. Such was the case
for Gail. She had a dream of her childhood home where

she lived with her now-deceased mother until she was fourteen years old. In the dream she felt the same warmth and love from her mother as she did when she was alive. In this case, the dream was experienced not as a letting go, but as a confirmation that her mother was part of the new life growing inside of her. She was not saying good-bye to a part of her childhood but rather integrating a facet of motherly love she thought she had lost forever. She realized from her dream that even though her mother was dead, she was still her baby's grandmother, and a connection could be maintained over time and space. The recurring presence of her mother in her pregnancy dreams helped Gail feel calm and confident even though it was her first baby. She never felt the level of anxiety about the birth process common among women giving birth for the first time. She was guided by the memory of her mother.

Some dreams of the past very clearly express to a mother-to-be that it is time to let go of old things and get ready for the wave of change that is sweeping in new life. Such was the case for Hope. In her dream, the past was literally embodied by certain articles she had possessed in San Francisco before she met her husband. As you will see, the specific items chosen by the unconscious are not devoid of humor:

> *I was on the beach in Malibu . . . not a place I go very often. There is a beach party going on. My ex-boyfriend is there but we are unable to connect. Strange things are coming in on the surf. A bookcase from Frisco, a pink hippie*

scarf also from Frisco, and finally a pair of underpants I recognize immediately . . . also from that period of my life. I try to collect my belongings, but the waves are not letting me do this. Suddenly I know that it is time to let that stuff go. I had some resistance because it was such personal stuff, but it is very clear that the ocean is allowing me to have a last look and that's it.

Upon looking at the dream more closely it became evident that Hope's unconscious had orchestrated the dream masterfully. First off, it was impossible for her to connect with her ex-lover, a definite sign that it was time for her to move on. Then there were the items that washed up on the shore. The bookcase stood for a time in Hope's past when she was exploring new ways of thinking and living; at this point in her life she was going to school and enjoying a greater sense of freedom than she ever had before. The pink hippie scarf was like a gauzy memory of life unencumbered by adult responsibilities, such as marriage and children. It infused her with a sense of youthful beauty; Hope felt pretty wearing it. The underpants that came in on the waves were an intimate reminder of the sexual freedom and experimentation she went through at that time. So you see, the message of the dream is concrete and direct. It leaves no room for doubt. It shows clearly that a new phase of life is about to begin. It is time to say good-bye to the past. It can be looked at and mourned, but don't hang onto it.

● ● ●

The desire of the psyche to make room for the new is expresssed just as effectively and directly in the following dream. This dream also happens to be a literal request for more space:

> *I am in our one-bedroom apartment. My baby is all swaddled, lying on top of the TV set. There is no space to put her anywhere else. I am holding her with my index finger. I can't do this forever. It's ridiculous. It's obvious that we need more space for the baby.*

At the time of the dream, Alexis had actually begun to look for a new home that would include a separate room for her baby. The above dream was s confirmation that she indeed needed to create space for her new child and that her old apartment was insufficient. In the dream, Alexis's index finger is not only holding the baby, but also pointing at it. It's as if the baby is saying "Look, here I am, make room for me." On the same note, 90 percent of the women we interviewed were in the process of looking for a bigger home or moving into a new one during their first, second, and even third trimester. Anybody would think that being pregnant is the worst time for such a move (think big boxes and heavy furniture), but when a woman is preparing to give birth to her child, certain nesting instincts take over, manifesting both in the mother-to-be's dreams and in real life.

Dreams of Lost Love

Dreams of "lost love" or former lovers are another important aspect of dreams of the past. In order for a woman to make room for the new life she is carrying, she has to have some closure with unfinished or old relationships. There are two categories in this realm. The first one has to do with mourning the loss of what could have been, the "what ifs" of life. What if I had married Jeff instead of Mark? What if I had accepted his invitation to his country home, etc.? The unconscious mind revisits these fantasies in dream time to finish stories that were left incomplete in the heart and mind of a pregnant woman. It is a cleansing cycle necessary in order to make room for the newly conceived child. It is an area of background baggage, a sort of lost-and-found of the psyche, wherein old material is processed so that new depths of love may be reached. A woman's pregnancy is the catalyst for such a clearance.

The second category of dreams involves past relationships and significant former lovers. These dreams can be a little more ruthless. Several women we interviewed had dreams in which their old lovers were killed off. In these cases, the women's psyches were making a harsh break between the past and the future. On an unconscious level they were exterminating old forms of love so that they could have more psychic space in which to care for their child. Both Karine and Tracy— two women we interviewed—had a series of dreams in which their ex-lovers became injured or died. In their waking lives, they had not even been thinking of these men, but in their subconscious memory banks, the cleansing process was well under way.

Tracy's dreams of the past were particularly interesting in that they included all of her ex-lovers, her stepfather, and even her husband. They all got killed off in her first trimester. Clearly, Mother Nature, the feminine principle of life, was taking over and making a clean sweep of all male energies. These inner characters had become superfluous; they were not necessary for the successful creation of a baby. The amount of rage present in Tracy's dreams was another manifestation of the power of Nature. In her sleep she was consumed with anger toward her husband, and she also believed her husband to be charged with a similar rage toward her. These feelings were so vivid in her dreams that she often woke up and had to ask her husband if he was angry at her. Of course, he said no. Still, she was astounded by the intensity of the feelings expressed in her dreams during that time. Fortunately this pattern of rage subsided by the end of the first trimester, and her dreams became more even keeled.

(One noteworthy exception in the murderous trend of Tracy's early pregnancy dreams was the harmonious connection with her ex-lover Derek. In real life he was the only one who had made the difficult transition from lover to friend. And in her dreamscape, he remained that faithful friend, someone she could count on and trust. Derek represented the type of safe male energy she wanted to keep around while her body was getting used to its new duties.)

Lynda was another interesting case. She is the mother of three boys all under the age of four. During all her pregnancies, she had recurring dreams of an ex-boyfriend she had loved for many years. "He was bad for me," Lynda said. "But I loved him so much I thought

I would die when it was over." Consciously, Lynda thought her ties with this man had been broken a long time ago, but her unconscious believed otherwise. There was a lot more letting go to be done. It took all three pregnancies for him to be cleared from her psyche.

Lynda's dreams showed her repeatedly that he was not interested in her anymore. He ignored her or treated her like a stranger in all the dreams she had of him. Her psyche was making it clear to her that the relationship was over. She could not believe that she was still dreaming of him while carrying her third child. So many years had passed. But she was relieved to find out that during her final pregnancy the dreams were not so intense or long. "I only had a few dreams," said Lynda. "And they weren't as vivid or disturbing as the first two pregnancies. It was as if he was fading away."

Another variation we found in the dreams relating to ex-lovers was in Jenny's dream of a fire station. When she walked into it, there was a party going on. A fireman she had dated in real life was there, and he asked her permission to walk her outside to her car so that she could go home. It was a very dark night and quite scary. In this case, the past, in the guise of the fireman, was symbolically escorting her to her new life. She was getting a nice send-off party. It was a celebration. But the journey she was embarking on was still scary and no one from her past could come with her. The fireman didn't get killed off, but she had to say good-bye to him and get into her car alone and do her own driving. This is Nature's way of saying, "Certain aspects of your old life are over. It's time for you to become a mother."

When many women become pregnant for the first

time, there is a feeling of "no turning back," "this is for real." Terminating old relationships through dreams of the past is the psyche's way of dealing with the new evolution of a woman's life. It is the way the soul prepares for tomorrow.

Dreams of the past are a powerful expression of a woman's inner desire to become as whole and free as she can to bear a healthy child. They are, if you will, the psychological equivalent of a woman's concern for her own physical well-being. For example, a woman quitting smoking and/or drinking and eating more healthfully when she becomes pregnant carries the same force as a dream of the past. Although the former are voluntary actions and the latter is subconscious, all are similar attempts made by the soul to prepare a woman for motherhood.

If a woman follows through with the guidance she receives from a dream of the past, she will greatly affect the relationship between herself and her child. A new bond will be created, one in which the patterns of the past no longer have an adverse effect on the present.

We have all heard of the sensitivity of unborn babies to loud noises, arguments, music, etc. This sensitivity also exists at a level of consciousness. When a dream of the past occurs and a woman responds to it consciously, the baby can feel the shift in the mother's awareness. It is as if the psychic link between the mother and child is suddenly more clear. This happens because the mother is responding to the flow of Nature; she is yielding to the natural cycle of healing in which the past is drawn into the present for clarification and analysis. When a mother ignores this process, her relationship with her child becomes burdened by projections. The past clouds the present and prevents the two souls from meeting each other with unhindered closeness.

What is natural is for the mother's childhood issues to surface, as well as any and all important relationships that she has experienced in her life. This is Nature's way of preparing the woman for motherhood. The more lingering feelings from her past a woman can resolve through her dreams, the more room she will have for the child, not only in her body but in her heart and mind as well. It is a simple equation. There must be some measure of peace about the past in order to freely embrace the future.

EXERCISES

Healing Childhood Dreams

The following exercises are meant to assist the mother-to-be in becoming more aware of what childhood feelings or old relationships are coming to the surface through her dreams. They are based on the first trimester and show the woman how to integrate these nightly experiences into the present landscape of her pregnancy.

Before Going to Sleep

Turn off the lights. Lie comfortably on a flat surface, with all limbs untangled, in an open and receptive posture. Close your eyes. Breathe once or twice deeply. Let go of tension. Pay particular attention to your neck and shoulders, to your jaw, and to your stomach; these are all areas where anxiety and worry can build up, often undetected. Feel your worried mental chatter fade away as if someone was turning down the volume of a radio until it is completely inaudible. Be aware of your beating heart pumping blood, not only for yourself, but also for the other life being created at this very moment in your womb. You are in the process of creation right now. You are the embodiment of life itself. Allow the womb of life to hold you as your own womb holds your baby, safely. Be aware that everything that has ever happened in your life has led you to this moment here and now. Be in the present and know that all of your life is contained in this moment. All of your life experience is available to you right now. All of the wisdom of your ancestors is available to you right now. Feel their support.

In this receptive stillness, ask your unconscious to reveal to you the places in yourself where love is lacking, where there is an emotional knot that needs to be untied so that life can flow, where space needs to be made for the new life that is emerging. Trust that your dreams will lead you safely where you need to go, and let sleep nourish both your body and your soul so that you, in turn, may nourish the life of your unborn child.

After You Wake Up

Take your time transitioning from sleep to being awake. Let the images from your dreams drift into your consciousness unimpeded by the concerns of your daytime responsibilities. Be still with your thoughts. Let the dreams surface to the forefront of your conscious mind.

If you are confronted with a dream from the past, let the landscape and the characters tell you what they mean. Ask them and yourself these questions:

- What are you doing in my dream? What are you trying to show me or tell me?
- Do I need to tell these characters how they make me feel? Was something left unsaid or undone?
- What do I need from the characters in the dream, if anything?
- How do I feel in the dream? Did something happen that bothered me?
- If I could, would I change the ending or even the whole story?
- How? What would I say or do? What would the other characters say or do?

Give yourself time to hear the answers and allow yourself to be surprised. Write them down if you think you will forget them. Then proceed to the next step: reliving the dream but changing the ending or outcome so that the resolution is more harmonious and creates peace of mind. You can even change the reactions of the characters involved. Create your ideal scenario. You are the producer, director, and screenwriter, not to mention the actor of every part. I recommend doing the exercise twice. Often new elements appear at the second go-around that were overlooked the first time.

Begin by re-creating and reliving the dream as completely as possible, remembering the feelings that went along with it. Once you feel that you are fully entrenched in the world of the dream, start to guide the dream into new directions that feel more satisfying, more healing. Bestow a different tone to the landscape. Select new reactions and new words for the characters. Make yourself the heroine of your dream. Give yourself what you need to feel successful or safe or simply more whole by the end of the dream.

The dream is offering you something to look at in your own psyche, a challenge if you will. "This is the stuff you carry in your body and in your mind. What should you do with it? Do you want to keep it, dump it, integrate it?"

When you actively engage your dream in this way and bring it to a satisfying conclusion, you have answered the call to bring your consciousness up to date. You are participating in your own healing and providing a safer psychic space for your child to grow in. You could call it "spring cleaning for the psyche" or "clearing the cobwebs from the past." It certainly gives a hint or even a push to your unconscious mind to keep clearing the old and making room for the new.

You can apply this procedure to dreams concerning childhood issues as well as ones involving old love and relationships. What you want to keep in mind in dreams involving past relationships is that the people you were intimate with played a role in your evolution as a human being. You were with them for a very good reason: to learn something, to let go of something, etc.

Sometimes such dreams of the past are about unfinished business, in which case the above exercise will be extremely useful, so that you may give your story with that person a satisfying ending.

The other thing to keep in mind is that the love you felt for those people is real, and that *love is never lost*, even if the person is out of your life forever. In fact, all we are ever learning to do is love well. When you accept that the love is yours to keep, not only do you expand your capacity to love, but you also free up the love that was stored in your mind, in the knots of your body, and make it available to yourself and others who are ready to receive it now. Love is love. It is the other feelings we surround love with that need to be let go of, to be healed.

CHAPTER TWO

The Second Trimester: Dreams of Bonding with the Child

If the dreams of the first trimester revolve mostly around letting go of the past, the dreams of the second trimester seem to center around the bond that is being established between the unborn child and the mother. At this point, the relationship is more tangible and the dreams start to include both the mother and child in various dynamics. The sense that a genuine human being is developing inside the womb is played out in the dreamlife, preparing the woman for the later stages of pregnancy and finally the birth itself.

Most second-trimester dreams fall under three general categories. One category involves anxiety dreams, which usually have to do with the woman worrying about whether or not she is going to be a good mother. This is especially prevalent among women who are becoming parents for the first time. In their dreams, they might find themselves afraid of misplacing their baby or not liking its appearance, for example. Anxiety dreams can take on a multitude of forms, but usually have one thing in common: They leave the mother-to-be distraught and nervous about the condition of her child. She wakes up unsettled and can remain fearful unless she understands that the dream is helping her adjust to motherhood by processing her unconscious fears.

Another category of second-trimester dreams involves the time when mother and child begin to see each other in dreamtime. It is again an opportunity set forth by the unconscious, creating a bond between the two beings that is clear and vital. In some dreams, the skin of the mother's belly actually becomes transparent and stretchy, like a window through which she is able to view her baby. In other dreams, the mother is able to take the baby out of the womb and put it back in at will, experiencing for brief moments what it feels like to be two separate entities alive in the world.

In the third category of dreams, mother and child become part of the natural world. They can take on animal forms, (the baby shifts shape more often than the mother) and experience each other in a way that transcends human dimensions. In these dreams, the setting often includes watery landscapes: oceans, lakes, and caves. The mother-and-child scenario goes through all sorts of wild variations: The child might appear to the mother as a kitten or a puppy. During this time in the pregnancy, all sorts of dreams are possible. The unconscious mind is more active than usual, flooding the woman's sleep with strange and mystical adventures.

One thing is for certain: The dreamscapes of the second trimester are not boring. They are often fraught with anxiety and fear, because it is at this time in the cycle of her pregnancy that a woman must develop a sense of responsibility for another human being. She is no longer just carrying a small embryo. Her child has taken form and the birth is now an approaching reality.

Anxiety Dreams

Several women I interviewed toward the end of their second trimester had dreams of giving birth too early. In their sleep, they usually tried to get the baby back inside the womb because they knew instinctively it was not ready to be born. There is a direct correlation between this type of dream and the physical development of the baby. If the baby were to be born at this time in the pregnancy, it would need an incubator to survive, and even though the woman is asleep, she knows this to be true.

One of these women was so worried in her dream that her baby would be born too soon that she squeezed her thighs to keep her baby from falling out. The dream was so real for her that she woke up with intense muscle cramps between her thighs that took a couple of days to subside.

Fear of losing the baby can manifest itself in many different ways. Several women dreamed that their baby was so small they would misplace it and not even realize it had been lost. One woman dreamed that she was looking for something in the folds of white sheets but could not even remember what it was. She only knew it was very important to her and that she must find it.

I was in this white room with white sheets bunched together on a bed and I had to find "it," but I couldn't remember what "it" was or why "it" was so important to me. I just knew it was my responsibility. The anxiety I felt was so intense it woke me up.

This type of anxiety dream is nature's way of activating an involuntary mechanism in the mother to ensure the survival of the baby. What if a mother forgot or misplaced her child? What would happen to the baby then? Anxiety dreams, although they are not pleasant, send an important message to the parent. It is part of the process by which a woman becomes acquainted with the sense of duty and responsibility that comes with motherhood, and the reality of a baby's dependency on her for its survival. (This kind of dream is even more prominent in the first few months after the mother has given birth.) Women have reported hundreds of dreams in which they experienced the terror of losing or hurting their baby through drowning, dropping it, misplacing it, or forgetting where it was. The unconscious is hard at work making sure the mother is aware that the newborn cannot survive without her.

Many fears plaguing a pregnant woman are often difficult for her to admit to herself or talk about, which is one of the reasons why these fears have a tendency to be played out in the dreamscape. Several women we interviewed had dreams of not liking their baby or not being able to bond with it. Unconsciously, they were acting out their worst nightmares so they would not have to experience them in their waking life. In this case, dreaming becomes a way of exorcising fears, a soul-cleansing activity highly present in the second trimester. Jane, one of the women we interviewed, had such a dream:

> *I could see part of the baby sticking out. It was as if the skin of my stomach had disappeared. First I saw the foot of the baby, then its head. I couldn't believe what I was seeing. The head of the baby was that of a forty-year-old woman. She looked mean, like a school librarian who would tell you to keep quiet and report you to the principal if you didn't. She wore earrings and ugly, cakey makeup. Her hair was brown and lifeless. I decided to push the baby back in and reabsorbed it somehow.*

When Jane woke up and realized this was just a dream, she was very relieved. The idea of giving birth to a bitter old maid was not her idea of fun. But when we looked at her dream further, Jane saw that it was actually a gift. The dream enabled her to exorcise some of her fears about not liking her own baby. It also enabled her to deal with a part of herself she had not looked at before, an aspect of her feminine nature that was sad and lonely and acted with an authority she didn't feel.

The woman in the dream could also have been a reminder of other women in her family, perhaps a combination of her mother and her aunt. Taking in the gifts from the dream enabled Jane to embrace these aspects of her feminine self so that she could become more at peace with the idea of motherhood.

Very often such dreams will show that the

mother-to-be is resisting or even angry at the prospect of having a baby. But if she can look at her dreams with curiosity and compassion rather than judgment or fear, she will understand that her psychological development is running in tandem with the physical process of her pregnancy. In this way second-trimester dreams can help a mother-to-be to adjust psychologically to this earth-shaking physical transformation.

In second-trimester dreams, when the mother is in the process of bonding with her unborn child, the anxiety over becoming a mother or giving birth to an unlikely character is not always painful or sad but often full of humor and wit. The following dream is such an example:

> *In the dream I give birth to a plastic cowboy. He seems to be right out of the movie* Toy Story. *He is about six inches tall. He tips his hat to me and swings his lasso. I stare at him, dumbfounded. I wake up laughing. He reminds me of my husband.*

The dreamer could not get over the wildness of her imagination. She thought that she had stepped into a cartoon. The little toy cowboy was very cute and very determined to make his presence felt. He was the one in charge of the bonding process with his mother and he had literally taken her heart with a lasso. He also had the unmistakable swagger and energy of his father. The dream's playful quality greatly helped the mother-to-be get over her fears about her baby's health. The baby became very real to her with a definite personality full of vim and vigor.

• • •

One type of anxiety dream occurs more often with older women. It usually happens because women in their late thirties and forties are at higher risk for birth defects. An amniocentesis is therefore recommended in this case. In these women, anxiety dreams tend to take place during the waiting period before the mother-to-be gets the results.

The following dream is fairly typical and encapsulates the fears a woman has of not giving birth to a healthy child. This kind of dream is quite different in tone from the more humorous dreams in which a woman gives birth to a kitten or a full-grown human being or some other strange species.

> *I am in a classroom with other mothers and their babies. My baby is brought in. He is physically perfect but only three inches long. He never matured and he will never grow up like the other babies. I am devastated. My heart breaks. I worry whether the other children will tease him or ever play with him.*

This was a very difficult dream for Alexis. It conjured up feelings of worry about her amniocentesis and what she would do if the doctor told her her baby will have abnormalitites. Fortunately, Alexis never had to make that type of decision because she had a healthy baby, but the dream helped her ask herself some tough questions and clarify her motives for having the amniocentesis. After she woke, Alexis wondered why she had the test in the first place, for her benefit or the child's.

This dream exorcised fears for her that she had not been completely conscious of.

Bonding Dreams

Instead of being an exorcism, sometimes a second-trimester dream can be a benediction and provide answers to deeply held fears. This was true for Karen. During her first pregnancy she started to worry a lot about whether or not she would be a good mother. By the time she reached her second trimester, this worry had become an obsession. She didn't know what to do about it until she had the following dream:

> I am looking at my baby and she is looking back at me with a big smile. There is so much trust in her eyes. She is reaching with her arms toward me. She seems to be telling me that I'm trust-worthy. I wake up feeling that the dream is an answer to a prayer. It comforts me on the deepest level. It was as if my baby had told me that everything would be okay.

After that dream, Karen was able to go through the rest of her pregnancy without worrying about her abili-ties as a mother. She started communing with her unborn child and allowed herself to be present with what was happening, rather than worry about what might be. The dream had been a transforming agent, taking her through the arduous trials of the second trimester into a confident birth.

The bonding dreams of the second trimester take on an added dimension when they are coupled with an image from the past. The mother is then able to grasp more fully the impact of the impending birth. Susan felt a strong connection with her unborn child, but it wasn't until she experienced the following dream in her second trimester that its implications became real for her. She had just finished taking a grief workshop when she had this emotionally stirring dream:

> *I am in church listening to the choir singing. I am holding an oil painting of my father's face. I am looking straight into his eyes. I am over-whelmed with grief as I realize that he will never meet my baby and my baby will never meet his grandfather. I start to sob in the dream. I wake up with tears running down my cheeks. I am still crying.*

The grief work Susan had done, combined with this stage of her pregnancy, had crystallized in this dream of loss. The reality of her baby's existence made the reality of her father's death more poignant. By the same token, her father's death also affected her awareness of the baby's life. This dream was very cathartic for Susan and it helped her deepen her bond with her unborn child even more.

Another type of dream that occurs during the second trimester centers around the baby being taken away or growing up too fast. This is the double bind of the mother-to-be. On the one hand, Nature is preparing the mother to become fully responsible for the survival and well-being of her new child, and on the other hand, she is being instructed ahead of time that this baby does not belong to her and will grow up sooner than she thinks. These are tough dreams for a woman to have, even when they are full of humor, and usually leave the mother with the feeling that some things are beyond her control.

The context for these dreams varies. Sometimes in the dream the baby grows up the minute it comes out of the womb, turning into a toddler or even a fully grown adult. In other dreams, the child is born already fully grown, with facial hair and adult mannerisms.

These dream sequences are very much a part of the collective unconscious—the part of our psyche that is connected to our fellow human beings as a whole; in other words there is the individual psyche and the collective psyche. They pop up in certain oral traditions, like the African version of one of these stories, in which a baby comes out all grown up and gives his mother a lot of trouble. Coincidentally, one of the pregnant women I interviewed had read this story to her third graders when she herself was in her second trimester. She realized how similar to her own deams this fairy tale was. This is what she dreamed:

> I had a series of dreams in which my baby grew up at an unreasonable rate. It really upset me after all I had been through to have him. In one dream he went from infant to toddler in an instant. He started running from one person's lap to another at a party, growing all the time. In another dream, my baby grew up in one day, all of a sudden. He went from being an infant to

an adult. I never got to enjoy any of it. I woke up disconcerted and rather mad, like someone had played a bad trick on me.

All these dreams of the second trimester are a way for the mother-to-be to start dealing with the reality of what is to come. They are tools the woman can take advantage of to work through her fears about becoming a mother. Some of these dreams are really not so much anxiety dreams as bonding dreams. The mother gets a chance to commune with her future baby without having to deal with the actual raising of the child. These dreams can be very magical and yet feel very natural at the same time. One of Dayna's dreams shows this very well:

This dream happened several times during my second trimester in one form or another. I guess you could call it a recurring dream. I can see the baby through my stomach. The skin is so translucent and stretchy, the baby is able to grab my finger through the skin of my stomach. She takes my finger and wraps it around like babies do, real tight. Sometimes the baby pushes her foot out so I can see it and even hold it. It's wild. Actually, it's really a thrilling experience and I feel happy to be able to touch my baby before she is born.

Then once in a while I have a dream where something even more amazing happens. I can actually take my baby out of my stomach and then put it back in at the end of the day. I even take her to the mall and she doesn't cry or anything. The

*only thing is that she cannot be touched by any-
one else yet. She is not ready for that.*

These were wonderful dreams for Dayna. She
laughed after recounting them because in some ways
she knew this was the easiest time she would ever have
with her baby. As another woman told me, "The baby
is with me everywhere I go, but it's all self-contained.
No carriage, no diapers, no crying. It's ideal. I feel completely content." You can tell these are women in the
second trimester. The nausea and discomfort of the first
trimester are over and the physical discomfort of the
third trimester has not yet set in.

Therefore, even though the second trimester can be
full of anxiety dreams, it is also a time when the exqui-
site symbiosis between mother and child is at its peak.

Animal Dreams

The dreams of the second trimester are also the arena
for some interesting interactions with the "wild
kingdom." Many women seem to be in touch with the
natural aspect of pregnancy through their connection
to animals. Some of these connections can be to pets
they own and some are with animals in the wild. In
these types of animal dreams, the woman is usually
taken out of her regular "human" surroundings and
placed in the habitat of the animal she is dreaming of.
Sometimes she will be in a tropical forest, sometimes in
the ocean, communing with seals, for example.

If there is a metamorphosis, it is usually the unborn child who will be changed into an animal. (This makes sense as it is the child who is growing into a human being.) This theme of the transformation of a child into an animal is also a part of the collective unconscious and pops up in many fairy tales. The baby in these stories is usually called "the changeling" and often possesses unearthly powers that scare the people around him.

Of course, there are always exceptions to the rule. We found at least one woman who related a dream in which she saw herself as a female cougar with her cub. In the dream she marveled at her strength and ability to protect her baby from anything and everything. The cougar represented the most natural, untamed, and fierce part of herself, the instinctual facet of her character, alive and ready for the upcoming birth. The woman felt a lot of respect and love for this animal. When she realized it expressed the instinctual, mother part of herself, she was in awe of its power and its beauty.

> *A female cougar is running around in and out of the forest with her cub. The onlookers seem to have a healthy respect for her. They know she is playing with her cub and seems very approachable, but the truth is, she is very fierce and would attack anyone who dared get too close to her offspring. I wake up feeling very emotional. There was something so majestic and real about the dream. It showed me an aspect of myself I didn't even know existed. Maybe it's true what they say about what maternal love can accomplish, like those amazing feats of strength and power.*

• • •

Most women who dream of adult animals in the second trimester tend to see the animal as female or representing a feminine aspect of life. It is as if the animal is educating the mother-to-be about the maternal forces of nature, how to raise their young, and the like.

One woman had consecutive dreams of swimming with dolphins all through her second trimester and well into the third. She felt as if she were swimming in an ocean of love. The nature of the dolphins was both playful and maternal. It reassured her, made her feel good about her pregnancy. On the cusp between the second and third trimester, the dreams with the dolphins literally took on a new depth. In the dreams, the dolphins were taking her down to explore a deeper part of the ocean. She was getting more and more acquainted with the creative force behind her own pregnancy. She was attuning herself to its rhythm, so different from her fast professional pace, a rhythm that involved listening to an ocean of life within her, a rhythm of blood pumping and organs being created. Sometimes she felt as if she were breathing underwater all the time, not just in her dreams with the dolphins, but in real life as well.

Marie also had recurring dreams of animals. Her dreams, however, centered around three or four white wolves who seemed to be protecting or guarding her. The dreams started at the end of her first trimester and proceeded into the second.

I am sleeping in the dream and at the same time
I am aware of the presence of these beautiful

white wolves. There are three or four of them. They are all around my body on the bed and even on top of me, but I can't really tell because I don't feel the weight of them, only their presence. I know they are here to help me but I'm not sure how or why.

In looking at her dream, Marie felt that the white wolves were symbolic of the protective, instinctual part of her nature. The wolves stood for both the wildness of the feminine and the mystery of what Marie was going through in creating a child. Marie expressed that she felt very well looked after in the dream, as if the wolves were her guardian angels.

Alexis dreamed of a horse during her second trimester. This dream stuck out in her mind because in real life she was incredibly allergic to horses. She had completely forgotten the dream until she went to the doctor to get the baby's heartbeat checked.

The doctor listened to the heartbeat of my baby, then turned to me with a big smile and said, "Your baby has the heartbeat of a horse." I nearly jumped out of the chair. I had just dreamed of a horse the night before and had promptly forgotten it. This horse was the color of chestnut with a luminous auburn and gold mane. The color reminded me of my husband's hair. I was absolutely in love with this horse, as if I had just given birth to it. I woke up feeling lighthearted and invigorated. It was a relationship I certainly never had to horses in real life, but it felt very real and very beautiful.

• • •

Upon looking more closely at the dream, we found that the horse in Alexis's dream was roaming free. It was proud, beautiful, and left her feeling strong. It was a very empowering dream. It expressed for her the energy and strength she felt making a baby and it reassured her as to the health of her child. This prognosis was confirmed very clearly by the doctor when he used the words "heartbeat of a horse" to describe the state of her baby's health. Her instinctual nature knew exactly what was going on with her baby and it was confirmed through the metaphor of the horse that the doctor used the next day.

In all the above dreams, the animals (whether they roam the earth or the depths of the ocean) stand for the instinctual, protective mechanism of Nature. They show the power of the feminine aspect of Nature, which is totally in charge at this time in a woman's life. The relationship a woman has to her instinctual nature is very important. Her level of comfort and her trust in it will be invaluable to her at the time of birth. If she can harness the strength and power of her own instinctual nature, as shown to her in her dreams, she can face the birth itself with more confidence and faith. She will feel more in charge of the whole process, or at least feel that she is working in tandem with Nature. This attunement to her own wildness will give her a sense of her own strength that she might not have if she only gives her trust to the medical machine.

Second-trimester dreams can be quite humorous in their depiction of mother and child. As mentioned earlier, it is usually the child, not the mother, who undergoes unusual transformations. Dayna's dream of her baby fits neatly into this category:

> *In my dream, my baby jumps out of my arms. I see it morphing into a cocker spaniel for some reason. The dog starts running around the kitchen and wagging its tail. l am stunned and I also want to laugh. I can't believe this is my baby.*

Dayna realized that the cocker spaniel was an animal that she really liked, something friendly and furry. This is what being pregnant with her baby felt like at the time—friendly. Many women relate to the unborn child as to a very dear pet right through the second trimester, especially if this is their first baby. Dayna's sister, Deedee, dreamed that she was nursing a kitten. Another woman dreamed that she found her cat, a calico, flat as a pancake under a mess of white blankets. She was very happy to find it again even if it was in an odd shape. She was greatly relieved since she thought she had lost it.

This same woman had expressed her worry about being able to love her baby as much as she did her cats. The dream encapsulated her fears perfectly. Of course, once the baby was born, she realized in an instant that her fears were completely unfounded. The depth of love she discovered within her was beyond anything she could have ever imagined. Motherhood unlocks this ultimate gift of unconditional love, which flows between the mother and the newborn. This love was at the essence of the following dream I recorded:

I am pregnant in the dream. A woman walks toward me. I remember seeing vivid colors. The woman hands me a ladybug. It has three black spots on it. Its texture is very velvety. It is the most precious gift I could ever imagine. I feel it in my heart. I wake up.

This woman considered the ladybug a precious gift. We agreed that the three spots on the bug probably expressed the time left until the baby was due, for she only had three more months to go. Delving further into the dream, we came to see that the ladybug was a symbol of love, much like a butterfly is a symbol of beauty and transformation, or a hummingbird, a symbol of dexterity, fragility, or joy. The ladybug holds the magic and beauty of life in its simplest, yet most precious form. It is no coincidence that several of the women we interviewed referred to their newborn as "my little bug."

Second-trimester dreams can help the mother and child to get acquainted on a deeper level. The woman is adjusting to her new size and shape and can turn her attention to the child growing within her. Her keen interest in her baby, its sex, its personality, is reflected in her dreams. If a woman allows herself to pay attention to her dreams during this time, she will see that a wealth of information is at her disposal. It is the kind of information that is not available in books because it is deeply personal, from the inside out. It is knowledge that comes from her own unconscious, her womb, and the baby within her, from all of her own matrilineal history stored in her mind and available in her nightly stories. If she allows it, her dreams can be her teachers and her helpers. They can show the mother-to-be her own instinctual wisdom and strength. She can establish a bond of trust and love with her child that will help them both at the time of birthing. For as a woman gives birth to a child, she also gives birth to herself as a mother.

EXERCISES

Bonding with the Child

These exercises are designed to assist the mother-to-be in maximizing the opportunities offered by her dreams during the second trimester. They are quite simple and focus mainly on the bonding process with the baby as well as the instinctual aspects of motherhood.

Before Going to Sleep

The second trimester is the time when you really begin to bond with your child. You can participate more fully in this bonding process by giving your unconscious mind tasks that will enhance your experience before going to sleep. When you are in bed, with the lights turned off, ready for sleep, relax by taking one or two deep breaths followed by very quiet breaths. Quiet breathing helps you become very focused and relaxed at the same time. It is the kind of breathing that occurs naturally during sleep. When you feel quiet and still within yourself, tune in to the child within. Allow your awareness to expand to include the dark and liquid space around this child, your own womb. Then allow yourself to be bathed in the darkness of the night. Be still, aware that you also are enveloped in the womb of earth, of night, of life.

In this state, give your unconscious some directives for your dreaming travels:

- I want to commune with my child more clearly.
- I want to find out more about who this baby is.
- I want to know what she/he needs to be healthy.

You can make up your own list or add to this one. You can ask for whatever you need to know or understand. But don't worry if you drift into sleep without giving your unconscious any directives; the fact that you attuned yourself to your child before sleep will affect your dreams accordingly.

After You Wake Up

When you wake up from a dream that stirred you emotionally, don't rush out of bed. Be still. Allow for some transition time so that you may gather information and remember details.

If you had an anxiety dream of some sort, look at the content and message of the dream. Ask the questions that the dream elicits from you:

- What information is my dream trying to convey?
- Do I need to look more closely at my feelings about this upcoming birth?
- What is familiar about the dream, what does it remind me of?
- What is unusual or foreign about it, what does it remind me of?
- Is there some action I can take to make myself feel more ready?
- What would bring me some peace of mind?
- Do I need more support from my husband, friends, medical team?

Once you have an idea what the answers to these questions are, write them down, always allowing room for more information to come through. The unexpected often carries great wisdom. This gathering of new images is nourishment for your psyche to expand upon, and ultimately will enhance the growing bond between you and your baby.

If you had an animal dream, determine whether you are a participant in the dream or a bystander. Did you change into an animal or did your child make the transformation? What kind of animal? If there is an adult animal in the dream it usually stands for an aspect of your instinctual nature. Ask yourself the following questions:

- What kind of animal is it?
- How do I relate to it? Do I like it? Am I scared of it or in awe of it?
- What energy does it convey?

If you decide that you like the energy of the animal but don't really feel that you possess its qualities in real life, do the following exercise.

You can perform the following steps before you get out of bed (it shouldn't take more than ten minutes).

When you are ready, close your eyes, take a deep breath to relax, and then engage in some quiet breathing. Bring up the image of the animal in your mind's eye. You can place it in the context of the dream if it helps your imagination. Make the image as clear and real for yourself as you can. Think of the coat of the animal, its color, the way the muscles move under the skin, its pace and speed, its strength, playfulness, wildness, and so on. Then ask yourself what it would feel like to have that pace, that speed, that kind of life force running through your body. What would it feel like to be this animal, completely in tune with yourself, your surroundings? How would this kind of strength feel?

Then take the next step and allow yourself to feel exactly what it would be like. Give yourself permission to move like a lion or howl like a wolf. Be a dolphin swimming and doing somersaults in the ocean. Feel what it would be like to have sonar, to be aware of sound vibrations from miles away. Feel the wildness and speed of a horse. Enter the realm of a mother lion protecting her cub. Of course, you are not a lion or a dolphin, but if you dreamed it, it is because the energy of the animal lives in you. Native Americans would say the animal is part of your "medicine." Being conscious of the energy the animal carries will allow you to tap into it when you need it, at the time of birth.

Once you have finished the exercise, it is useful to write down whatever information you have gathered as well as any other discoveries. The rational mind has a nasty tendency to invalidate experiences that stretch consciousness and embrace a more integrated view of life, where things are not so separate, so cut-and-dry.

CHAPTER THREE

The Third Trimester: Dreams of Impending Birth

During the third trimester, pregnancy dreams shift into high gear. The stage is set for the impending birth. The expansiveness of the dream themes of this last term reflect the round readiness of the mother-to-be. The Nature dreams often include tidal waves, earthquakes, or floods. There are waters overtaking dams and heavy rains soaking well-tended lawns. The imagery is vivid and powerful, a perfect mirror for the quickening in the darkness of the womb and the ripeness of the woman's body. In animal dreams, the cats, wolves, and horses of the second trimester are replaced by dolphins, whales, and elephants. The awesome power of Nature is displayed in all its greatness with these enormous animals.

At this time in a woman's path, everything in her body and mind is focused on the big event. The spotlight is on the star who is about to make his or her entrance into the world. The unconscious often interprets this image literally by including lots of star-studded dreams in the mother's sleep. Meryl Streep, Leonardo DiCaprio, and Brad Pitt have all appeared in the third-trimester dreams of many pregnant women.

For a woman to feel like a star at this time in her life makes sense, but sometimes she needs the fantasy of her dreamtime to feel sexy and desirable (which is not easy at eight or nine months of pregnancy), even if her husband reassures her that she is still the sexiest woman he has ever known. So dreams of sexy movie stars also represent an opportunity for a woman to express a sensuality that she might not be feeling every day with her sore back and swollen ankles.

Finally, third-trimester dreams are an opportunity for the pregnant woman to rehearse the birthing process itself. Some women I interviewed dreamed of giving birth over and over again until the actual birth took place. Besides allowing for all sorts of wild scenarios to take place and hidden anxiety to be expelled, third-trimester dreams are also a wonderful way for a woman to get in touch with the reality of what is about to happen, sometimes in a matter of days or even hours.

Dreams of Nature

During the third trimester, dreams of Nature take on a more fearsome quality. There is a sense that everything is being overrun by the creative power of life. The waves are higher. The currents are stronger. The rivers spill over dams and turn towns into lakes. At this time a woman often feels like she is ready to burst. She feels both waterbound and earthbound, as if all she'll ever wear are tents and shoes that are one size too big.

Lisa's dream is one such example in which the power of Nature is obviously at hand. There is an additional element that clearly conveys her need for her husband's support at this time. This adds a dimension of poignant reality to the dream.

> *I am in a town where the water is beginning to rise. I know that nothing can stop this flood from happening. We are watching it all unfold from the edge of the town, near a forest. The town is becoming a lake and there is nothing I can do about it. It's quite terrifying to watch . . . and fascinating at the same time. I really need my husband Tom to come and help me, but I can't find him. There is a kitten floating on the water that I want to save. I'm desperately trying to get Tom's attention, but I can't. Eventually he understands how important this is to me and helps me rescue the kitten. He actually works really hard to get it out once he makes the commitment. I am very happy that the kitten is safe. It got a little squished in the process, but it's fine. I wake up feeling relieved, but it was a very intense dream.*

Looking at the dream together, we saw that Lisa was overwhelmed by the idea of giving birth to her second child on her own. She was afraid that her toddler would be lost in the shuffle. In real life, she had not felt supported by her husband in her previous birth. In fact, during her first pregnancy her husband had suffered from tremendous anxiety and a debilitating depression. She didn't want to go through this again.

In the dream, Lisa has no control over the flood that is "turning the town into a lake." In other words, eventually she will have to give birth. There is nothing she can do to stop Nature's process. However, she has some control over how she deals with the event. In the dream it is quite clear that she does not want to go through the experience alone. She keeps calling out to her husband to help her and she does not stop calling until she gets his attention. Eventually he responds and rescues the kitten. This turned out to be true in real life. Lisa's husband was able to be very present and emotionally available for her second birthing. In the end she felt that he had really helped her just as he did in the dream.

Another dream that involves a loss of control or surrender to the elements of Nature shows us how getting ready for the birth process is in itself a journey back to the origins of life. In the following dream Mina finds herself caught in the rain with her husband:

> *I am with my husband in the car. It is pouring rain. We are going to the hospital so that I can deliver my baby safely. I am not in pain even though I am in labor already. Suddenly the car stalls. It won't start again. It is flooded. The rain is coming down harder and harder. I remain fairly composed, but my husband is in a panic. He tells me I have to walk to the hospital and he will stay with the car. I get very angry at him. This is completely unacceptable. He looks*

sheepish, so I calm down. He finds some kind of a cart with one wheel and handles. It looks old and rickety. I climb in, not feeling too glamorous. I am drenched, soaked through. He is pushing me down the road. I think to myself that if I was not in labor, I would find this very funny. The hospital is on top of a hill. The hill is vast and with a well-manicured lawn. We start to cross the lawn, but it has turned to mud and we just can't go any further. I climb out, sit in the mud, and plant my feet firmly in the earth. It becomes clear to me that I will never reach the hospital and this is where I am supposed to give birth. A woman wearing a long emerald green cloak arrives from the direction of the hospital. She is my midwife. I wake up feeling strangely relieved in spite of the fear and anxiety I experienced in the dream.

Mina's dream is very significant for several reasons. To begin with, the rain plays a powerful role. It literally stops the plans of the couple to have a hospital birth and instead forces Mina to give birth in the muddy grass. There is something primordial about the mud. This is where the first signs of life appeared, the place where earth and life-giving waters mixed together. Though it is not a very comfortable place to give birth, Mina believes she has arrived at the right location. The midwife is an interesting character in that she comes from the direction of the hospital but does not necessarily belong to it. She is also wearing a green cloak of a rich color. Green is the color of spring and new life, particularly significant in the context of the imminent birth.

This dream also mirrors the conflict Mina had with her husband about whether to have a natural birth with a midwife or a regular birth in a hospital. The solution to the couple's dilemma is also part of the dream: to have the birth with a midwife who is connected to a hospital and to have the hospital close by in case of emergency.

Finally, the role of the husband in the dream is quite significant. At first he is reluctant to abandon the car, which is a modern mode of transportation and a safer way to travel. He has to push his wife in an old cart, a much more primitive mode of travel, which actually turns out to be the more effective tool in this situation. Again the dream shows Mina that entering the birthing process is entering the ancient mystery of life. Modern conveniences cannot take you through it, no matter how helpful they are. The active, rational side embodied by the figure of the husband in the dream has to be willing to be of service to the feminine. Husband and wife must work together, but Nature is in charge.

Upon further exploration, Mina found that the dream left her with a better understanding of the landscape she was entering and how to handle the birth itself. It exorcised some of her anxiety about not getting to the hospital on time. She also felt more compassion for her husband who was trying to protect her in the best way he knew how. When Mina shared her dream with her husband, they were able to come to an agreement: They decided to go for a home birth, but maintain a rapport with a hospital in case of emergency.

Mina's husband admitted that he had had dreams of his own about not getting to the hospital in time. These dreams left him feeling completely overwhelmed and out of his depth about the birth. Accepting the enormity of the event was a relief for both of them.

Sharing the feelings this dream brought to the surface had a profound impact on both husband and wife. It helped them acknowledge their individual needs and fears about the birth. The dream also got them in touch with the meaningful mystery of bringing new life into the world in a way nothing else could have.

Such dreams of Nature are part of the initiation into motherhood pregnant women go through, culminating with the birth itself. When birth is imminent, nature dreams show the woman that it is time for her to surrender to the inevitable conclusion of the gestation period. The seemingly cataclysmic events depicted in these dreams are different from the ones caused by the hormonal turmoil of the first trimester; in this instance, they render an accurate depiction of what mother and child are about to experience emotionally and physically. The dreams show the woman that becoming one with the rain, the mud, or the flood is a way for her to "embrace" rather than "brace herself against" the forces at play during birth. These dreams can be a wonderful psychological tool for the mother to use as part of her preparation for the birth.

Animal Dreams

Many of the women interviewed during their third trimester had entrancing dreams in which dolphins and whales were prominently displayed. Contrary to the

Nature dreams, there was nothing particularly threatening about these mammals. It was often a dance of joy the women witnessed and shared with the babies in their wombs. Some of the women felt so connected to these animals that they expressed an urgent desire to go swimming with them in the ocean.

In Native American tradition, the dolphin embodies the breath of life. It evokes the rhythm and energy that is present in all of existence. It is the life force in its purest form, the manna or mother.

Legend has it that the moon instructed the dolphin to live with this rhythm of life. It is the very same rhythm or cycle that women experience during their menstruating years. When Dolphin learned the rhythm of life, he was able to enter the dreamtime and discover true communication, a multileveled world of sound and pattern.

Dolphin did not know what to do with this knowledge when he returned to the ocean until Whale told him that he could become the messenger between the children of earth and the dwellers of the dreamtime, the very ones who knew Great Spirit. Women who dream of dolphins are touching the core of this pulsating breath of life. They know through the dreamtime that they are the source, the giver and the recipient of life. It is a joyful and thrilling experience that often occurs in the second trimester as a subtle call to the deeper rhythms of Nature and finds its fruition in the third trimester as the breath of life.

When it comes to Whale, it is she who holds the ancient records of Mother Earth's history. People who have what Native Americans call "whale medicine" are very close to Great Spirit. They know things and have no idea why or how they know what they know. They can often hear things that no one else can. What people commonly refer to as "feminine intuition" is an aspect of whale medicine, and never is a woman more intuitive and open to subtle vibrations or frequencies than at the time of her pregnancy. Like Dolphin, the gift of Whale is wordless communication. It is an emotionally balancing and soothing tone that comes from Great Spirit.

When women meet with Whale or Dolphin in their dreams, they are opening themselves to the primordial rhythms of nature, to the principle of creation they so clearly embody during their pregnancy. It is often a moving, even emotional encounter, not only because women are in awe of the majesty and beauty of these mammals, but also because these mammals are a reflection of the deep rhythms of life that run most strongly through all women at the time of giving birth.

In the following example, the dream of whales is closely related to the woman's perception of her inner life and how this perception has been transformed by the imminent birth of her baby.

> I am 7½ months pregnant in the dream, which is exactly what I am in real life. I am standing by a lake. There are other people around. We are on a vacation of some sort together. Looking over the lake, although I don't see anything, I become absolutely convinced that there are whales in the lake. I just know this without knowing how I know it. I tell everyone about the whales. No one believes me. Suddenly two huge whales swim up by me. I tell "Luka," my baby,

to look through my tummy at the whales. He gets very excited. He recognizes them. Then I go to a mansion that is supposed to be my home. I've dreamed about this place before, but in the other dreams it was all run-down and dirty, and now it is clean and beautiful. I feel elated and serene at the same time. I wake up thinking this is the journey to my eternal heart.

The connection between the whales and the birth of the baby is made quite clear in the dream when Luka, the baby, sees the whales through the womb of his mother and recognizes them. Also, the mother is the one who knows the whales are coming. No one else believes it until they see them too. In other words, the mother-to-be is in tune with the wordless communication of her womb, which is getting ready for the birth.

The part of the dream that immediately follows the sighting of the whales reveals how the woman has been deeply changed by the growing baby in her womb. She visits a mansion that used to be "all run-down and dirty" and now has become "clean and beautiful." The simple beauty of this metaphor together with the sighting of the whales show how this woman has evolved and grown with her pregnancy. It has enabled her to sharpen her intuition, become healthier and more at peace with herself. A renovation of the spirit has taken place, symbolized by the clean beauty of the mansion. A confused young woman has been transformed into a woman who is aware of the magic and mystery of bringing life forth. She is a woman on a "journey to her eternal heart."

• • •

Dreams of dolphins held similar mystery and magic for another woman who had them during her second trimester right up until the end of the third trimester. One dream stands out among the other dolphin dreams. In it, she does not stay on the surface, playing and swimming with the dolphins as in previous dreams, but is taken underwater instead and into the birthing chamber. In this dream the dolphins show her that it is time to give birth. This is the last dream she remembers until she gave birth less than a week later.

I am on my back, resting on the ocean. I am so big my belly is keeping me afloat quite easily. A school of dolphins comes around me. I feel safe, protected by them. They know I am ready to give birth. I feel so honored to have this escort. One of them shows me the way down. I have to go with her. It's scary and I'm not sure I can do it. I manage to flip over. It's not very graceful. I feel like a large tub. My belly makes me sink down. It literally pulls me down under. The dolphin's presence next to me is reassuring. She guides me to an underwater cave. The cave is small, and even though it's dark, I feel that I am surrounded by starlight. Everything is shimmering. I shiver because I know this is where I have to go to give birth. The dolphin guards the cave's entrance. I wake up convinced I'm going to give birth now. In fact my labor starts two days later.

In this dream the dolphins take the mother-to-be down into the birthing chamber. The vivid image of her flipping over and her belly causing her to sink down to the bottom of the ocean perfectly mirror the changes going on in her body at this time: the baby turning upside down and dropping down low for the birth. This is very much a dream of preparation. And the relationship the woman has already established with the dolphins during the second trimester makes them the perfect escort into the final act of giving birth.

The underwater cave is the ideal location for the mystery of creation to unfold. In fairy tales, the cave is where treasures are found. The guardians of the cave are usually fearsome and test the hero before they allow her to enter. In this dream, however, the guardians are familiar guides whom the mother-to-be trusts enough to follow deep under the surface of the ocean in spite of her fear. Traditionally caves have been seen as the haven of a woman's sexuality, but in this dream they are much more than that. The cave shimmers with light, with the life that is about to be born into this world. It is a sacred dwelling. Like most dreams at this time of pregnancy, this one is infused with both the practical concerns of an imminent birth and the mystical qualities of life's greatest adventure.

In other parts of the world, whales and dolphins are less common than their earthbound counterparts, the great pachyderms of Africa and Asia. Elephants also appear in third-trimester dreams of women, not only as a symbol of the readiness of the mother-to-be, but also as a symbol of fertility, wealth, and wisdom. In India such dreams are considered a particularly great omen as the elephant represents the great elephant god known as Ganesha. Ganesha is a benevolent god who speedily brings good luck and prosperity. This god is also considered a good omen for the birth of a child, one who will bring honor and wealth to the household. In this sense, the elephant is not just a dream symbol, but is also invested with the cultural and spiritual beliefs of its country of origin.

Westerners have reported dreams of elephants during their pregnancy as well. The same rich imagery is available to them, but in most cases, for a westerner, an elephant is just an elephant, not a god. There is, however, a different kind of resonance in this symbol, which commands respect for its particular beauty and power. Like the whale, the elephant conveys a formidable presence, an awesome beauty that transcends aesthetics, and an endurance as old as life itself. It reflects the qualities of the feminine in a way that is beyond gender, theory, or philosophy. It is real, like an ancient memory, an anchor, a piece of earthly wisdom made flesh. It is a tremendous companion during labor if the woman can use it as an image to focus her attention. The elephant is a powerful symbol regardless of our cultural background. In dreamtime, the elephant might say to you, "Be like me, be the elephant during your birthing time. Trumpet your wild pain. Swing your body back and forth. Pour water over your body and cool mud on your aching back. My ancient wisdom is in your body also. We are one."

Dreams of great animals like the whale or the elephant in the third trimester are not only a signal to the mother that she and the baby are both ready for birth, but they are also a point of reference and an anchor for the mother-to-be to focus on during the birthing process. The woman's psyche is offering her dream images that are a powerful ally during the most painful parts of labor.

Our dreaming life is full of gifts, each one a perfect match for the moment we are living through. When we embrace the wisdom of our dreams, we bridge the gap between our waking and sleeping worlds in a manner that can enhance or resolve whatever situation or predicament we find ourselves in. When we harvest the underwater gifts of our nightly stories and bring them to the surface of our conscious mind, then the act of dreaming becomes part of our awakening to a richer life.

Star-Studded Dreams

Dreams of movie stars consistently appeared in the third-trimester dream world of the women I interviewed. When the movie star was a man, the mutual attraction between the star and the dreamer provided an opportunity for the woman to express her sexuality and to feel sexy. Sexual feelings can be very strong in dreams even though there is rarely any intercourse taking place. A woman in her third trimester can feel very sexy in her waking life, especially if her husband finds her pregnancy to be a turn-on, but if she does not, then her dreaming life provides a safe space for her to express that part of herself.

When the movie star was a woman, she often represented the dreamer herself, or at least some aspect of the woman that felt like a star at this particular time. In some cases, the star went through the labor on behalf of the dreamer, in a scenario reminiscent of the couvade syndrome that many men participate in in other parts of the globe. In couvade, the husband—usually with the help of the village elders—will act out the pain of the woman while she is in labor. The purpose of this is to distract any evil spirits from interfering with the birth and also to alleviate the woman's labor pains. This phenomenon is widely documented in Africa as well as the Caribbean and certain South American countries.

The following dreams were chosen because they include two stars that are dreamed about the most by pregnant women in their twenties. These two stars appear even if the women in their waking life are not great fans. The celebrities in question are Leonardo DiCaprio and Brad Pitt.

> *I am at a party in a house. I have been there before in previous dreams. I am hanging out with a bunch of movie stars, but the only one I am fascinated with is Leonardo DiCaprio. I think he is absolutely amazing. I am pretty sure he is in love with me, but actually I think I'm trying to convince myself of that. I am also quite aware that my husband is close by and that this would be an adulterous connection. Leonardo disappears in some other part of the house. I keep looking for him, going from room to room, but he is nowhere to be found. I don't feel a deep sense of loss because I know we are connected no matter what. I give up my search for now. I wake up.*

• • •

In discussing the dream with Lucy, she admitted to having quite a lot of celebrity-filled dreams during her third trimester. She was relieved to hear that she was not the only one and that these types of dreams were actually quite common in the third trimester. She told me that she was shocked to find herself attracted to another man while pregnant and married to a husband she loved. She also said that she felt very sexy in the dream—another common denominator in these kinds of dreams.

Lucy's connection to Leonardo DiCaprio does not end when she cannot find him. Even though he is not readily available, knowing that he is around is sufficient. The dream is simply showing Lucy that she is still a woman, still sexy even if she is about to become a mother. Even if she does not see it right now, she is still in touch with that part of herself. Her womanliness is still to be found even if it has to be relegated to the dream world right now.

During the third trimester, preparations for the baby's arrival are in full swing. Often the baby's room is made ready. There is a baby shower. The mother or sister of the pregnant woman might come to visit or stay until the birth of the baby. There are many events gravitating around the impending birth. There is also a joyous and anxious expectation, and a definite sense that the spotlight is on the woman who is about to take on the greatest role of her life. The woman may sometimes feel lost in the shuffle of intense activity devoted to the baby. She may need a space to live out her feminine fantasies, to feel desirable and sexy. The star-studded dreams provide such a haven.

• • •

This next dream is another example of a women's sexuality blossoming in her dreamscape during the last trimester. The woman mentioned that she had many dreams with celebrities in her last trimester, but this particular one stood out because it involved someone she had not had a crush on before, Brad Pitt.

> I am fooling around with Brad Pitt. He has his shirt off. I am totally crazy about him in the dream. I am definitely enjoying myself. I feel very attractive and very sexy. Nothing major happens, just a wonderful overall feeling of satisfaction and well-being. I wake up feeling sexy, which surprises me, considering I am huge at this point.

When the woman woke up, still feeling attractive and sexy, she realized the dream had played a very important role in changing her outlook. *Unattractive* is the word she had been using when referring to herself for the last couple of months. This dream, however silly or superficial it seemed, changed that. Her psyche had offered her a fun and lovely way of affirming and connecting with her sexuality. She grabbed onto it and her outlook improved. She started enjoying her pregnancy again in its last phase even though she had trouble getting around, eating, and breathing. She felt sexy, beautiful, and content in a way she had not experienced for a while.

Star-studded dreams not only help a woman explore and enjoy her sensuality, but they can also play a part in the rehearsal of the labor itself. This next dream illustrates this involvement perfectly. In it, a female movie star goes through the act of labor on behalf of the mother-to-be.

> *I am in labor in the dream. At the same time I am not the one actually giving birth to the baby. It's an odd sensation. I am observing my own labor performed by someone else. It turns out to be Meryl Streep. There is also a man with me in the room. He is supposed to be my partner. He is an actor. I think it's somebody like Jeremy Irons. Meryl Streep is the one experiencing my labor pains. When the baby comes out, it is a boy. As soon as the baby is out, I switch places with Meryl Streep. There is no doubt now that I am the mother. Meryl just went through the labor pains for me. I feel really honored and very lucky that she volunteered to endure my labor pains for me. I wake up.*

In our interview with the mother-to-be, we found out that Meryl Streep had been a role model for the young woman. She admired Meryl Streep as an actress and tried to emulate her acting abilities when she herself was an aspiring actress. She also thought of Meryl as a courageous human being, with strong ethics, good boundaries, and a great deal of common sense, all valuable qualities to have handy during labor. The dream provided Linda with a map to approach her labor. This map included all the qualities she had bestowed on Meryl Streep. The dream was telling her that she had a natural talent to go through this earth-shattering process. It showed her that she could be just like Meryl: a courageous, strong, and grounded person.

The French Lieutenant's Woman was also one of Linda's favorite films, which Jeremy Irons and Meryl Streep acted together. They were the perfect couple to show up in Linda's dream as the surrogate parents to her baby. More than that, Meryl Streep went through Linda's labor pains on her behalf, in a variation of the couvade ritual. In other parts of the world, this service is usually performed by the husband in real life, but here, Linda's favorite actress plays the role of the woman in labor. This dream allows Linda to get used to the labor itself in a safe way, while at the same time encouraging her to cultivate those qualities Meryl Streep possesses.

In star-studded dreams, the psyche is using a woman's unconscious connection to certain movie stars to express her sensuality, to remind her of her womanliness, and also to help integrate some of the qualities she has projected onto these people. All this is done in service of the mother-to-be, to assist her emotionally and physically through the last phase of her pregnancy.

The stars in the dreams also represent the feeling the pregnant woman has of being involved in a major production, playing a starring role in her life. This feeling is sometimes translated by a different kind of star-filled dream featuring a wedding. Although there are no celebrities in this case, the wedding itself can be considered the star-filled occasion. In such dreams, this symbol of birth becomes a newsworthy event, complete with lights and cameras.

On the eve of giving birth, mother and baby are the

center of attention, not only in their waking life, but in the dream world as well. Star-filled dreams for stars-in-the-making are one of the ways in which the psyche gets ready for labor.

Labor Dreams

With labor and delivery dreams the psyche attempts to assist the mother-to-be in preparing herself for the birth. In these types of dreams there is no couvade; the pregnant woman goes through the labor by herself. Most women experience recurring dreams of labor during their third trimester. Sometimes it is just the labor itself and sometimes it includes the delivery of the baby as well. As the woman gets closer to term, the dreams usually include both the labor and the delivery.

Dayna was no exception in that she had many rehearsal dreams of labor and delivery. These dreams included the car ride to the hospital. Her husband was the one who was driving her, as he would later in real life.

> *I am in the car with my husband. I am very calm and focused. I rehearse the rest of the labor in my head. I practice my breathing until we get to the hospital. Things go very smoothly. I am in the delivery room. Everything is very movielike. Everybody is doing what they are supposed to do. I am still calm. There is no chaos. Everything is very detailed. Then it is time to push, but I am not quite ready for that, so I wake up.*

One of the more interesting aspects of this dream was the atmosphere, which, Dayna insisted, was very calm and contained, not chaotic at all. The dream was very reassuring for Dayna and left her feeling that the birthing process would not be too overwhelming. Her dream was only giving her as much as she could handle. It stopped before the final phase of labor because she was "not quite ready for that."

When delivery time approaches, the dreams include not just the labor but the delivery as well. This happens more frequently for women who are pregnant with their first child. Somehow the psyche seems to know that there is no point in preparing a woman who has given birth once before. She will not be fooled by dreams of an easy delivery. She knows what it is going to be like.

As most women will admit, there is no perfect way to prepare for the journey of giving birth. You can take Lamaze classes. You can practice your breathing. You can read step-by-step instructions. You can study how many minutes apart the contractions will be during full labor. You can figure out how dilated you are. You can learn when you need to push. But each birth will still be unique, and have its own difficulties and miracles. Together the mother and child will cross into their own dimension where no one has gone before and no one can follow. The ones helping, the nurse, the doctor, the midwife, and the husband, are there to provide assistance, support, or even some relief in the form of the famed epidural, but there is no way they can know what the woman is going through. Only she does. Therefore, the psyche's way of helping a woman to prepare for labor and delivery is often to provide her with a reassuring dream image. Most dreams of labor and delivery are short and easy. The focus is on the joy at the end of the journey, the newborn child.

The next dream is no exception. The birth is easy, the bliss palpable. The psyche is using the dream as a medium to implant into the woman's memory the joy she will feel once the baby is born.

> *In my dream, the labor is quick. I can handle the pain. I am not overwhelmed. I think it's because of the method of birth I chose. I am giving birth in a bathtub. My child is born very easily. I sit up quickly when I feel his head pop out. I look at him. His eyes are wide open, even before he comes out all the way. Then I hold him immediately. It is the most wonderful sensation I have ever experienced. Beyond words.*

In real life, the woman had decided to give birth in a bathtub and this is reflected in the dream. There is a magical quality to the dream besides the easy birth: The baby is born with his eyes open. The most beautiful aspect of the dream, however, is probably the part the woman describes as "beyond words."

The gift of this dream is the experience of joy the woman feels when she holds her baby in her arms for the first time. This bliss-filled image is something she can really use to focus on during the delivery. This is the gift in most of the dreams of pregnancy at that time, and though it might misrepresent the labor, it is a powerful image for the woman to hold onto during her labor and delivery.

• • •

Labor is often represented in the dreamlife of the third trimester through traveling dreams, probably because giving birth is, metaphorically speaking, as foreign as traveling to another continent for the first time. In the following dream, the association between traveling and labor is made quite plain:

> We are in a motel. People come in to help me pack. I feel rushed, like I am on the run or escaping something, but there is no danger. The people tell us that we have to leave now and travel somewhere else. I can't quite catch the name of the place. It sounds familiar, but I have never been there before. Before we leave they ask me if I'm ready for some hard labor. I say that I can probably do it, but I would prefer it if they would ask my brother. He refuses, so it's up to me. I wake up.

The concept of travel in this dream is used in a very original manner. The woman is told in the dream that there is a rush, an urgency, which suggests that she is close to her due date. However, the traveling is not as important as the destination, which, she feels, is strangely familiar. The woman's unconscious knows the place she is going to even if she cannot remember its name. There is a memory that runs through all women, an ancient memory that links all female beings and has to do with giving birth. It is the other side of the coin. On the one hand the woman is going through this rite of passage alone because it is an experience unique to her. On the other hand, she is connected to all women who have ever been or will go through the act of giving birth. So it makes perfect sense that in the dream the woman would feel that her destination is both foreign and familiar at the same time. It truly is.

The next part of the dream is rather humorous, as dreams can often be. The people who are helping the woman in the dream ask her if she is ready to do some "hard labor." It does not take too much figuring out to realize that the dream is referring to her own imminent labor. The response is very honest. She would rather have her brother stand in for her but he refuses. The truth is, she must take this journey alone. In this dream the hard labor must take place before the woman can reach her destination, that is to say, before she can enter the next phase of her life. The hard labor in the dream symbolizes the gateway a woman has to go through before she becomes a mother.

This dream expresses in clear terms the idea that labor is a journey both strange and familiar, and that it requires hard work we would rather have someone else do for us if we had the choice. Couvade was probably born out of that desire. But our Judeo-Christian culture would be hard-pressed to accept such a concept.

Dreams of travel often incorporate various elements that add unexpected dimension to labor dreams. Such is the case of the following dream. In it, the mother-to-be is not only traveling, but also looking for "keys."

> *I find myself in London's Heathrow airport.*
> *When I get there I realize I shouldn't have flown*
> *because of the pregnancy. But no one realized I*
> *was pregnant. So I didn't have any problems. I*
> *feel fine. Traveling wasn't as bad as I thought it*

*would be in my condition. The airport is very
crowded. I am trying to find my sister and my
mom. I find their keys but not them. Then I
realize that I traveled to London in four hours,
as opposed to much longer. Actually it should
have taken me at least twelve hours or more, so
they probably aren't expecting me yet.*

The quick flight and unexpected arrival (the
mother and sister of the mother-to-be are not there)
all point to a premonition of a short labor, four hours
rather than twelve or longer. What is even more interesting in the dream is the fact that although the
mother and sister are not on the scene, the woman
finds their keys. What are these keys? In real life the
woman's mother and sister are both mothers. They
have both gone through labor and given birth. They
hold the "keys" to the experience of womanhood this
mother-to-be is about to enter. Even if they cannot be
there in the flesh, the fact that they have gone
through this experience and lived to talk about it is
helpful to the dreamer. The psyche recognizes the
validity of that help by having the dreamer find the
keys of her female relatives.

If giving birth to a baby can feel as strange as traveling to a foreign country, then it makes sense that the
unconscious mind would also create strange pictures of
the newborn baby. Labor dreams can be somewhat reminiscent of the anxiety dreams of the second trimester
when it comes to the delivery phase. Some women
dream of giving birth to aliens or some other unearthly
creatures, or even angels and devils. The truth is, a fetus

does look like an alien creature when you first see a picture of it. This type of third-trimester dream is also more common among younger women who are giving birth for the first time and have not had the relief provided by an amniocentesis.

One woman who experienced several dreams of giving birth to an assortment of ancient frozen creatures—aliens, angels, and devils—also dreamed that she gave birth to a baby who looked just like his father. This was as much of a surprise to her as her other more outlandish dreams. In this dream, the baby she had nurtured in her womb for nine months turned out to have nothing in common with her at all. The baby's appearance and personality reflected his father's only, not his mother's in the least bit. This can be difficult, even scary for a mother to accept, even if it is just a dream.

I am eight months pregnant when I have this dream. My baby comes out and immediately his father is holding him. The baby has his father's face. It's unmistakable. He has sharp dimples like his father with big eyes and brown hair. The baby has an older man's face. I am stunned. I did not expect my baby to look so much like his father and not at all like me. It is disappointing, but I know there is nothing I can do about it.

This same woman had several dreams of giving birth to a baby who did not look like her. She had other dreams where the baby came out looking quite alien, an ancient creature from another dimension. The woman's unconscious was trying to help her adjust to the fact that although she was bringing this new being into the world (after carrying it for nine months), it was different from its mother. It might even feel and look quite alien.

The next two dreams illustrate this notion of the baby's personal identity in a more radical fashion. They came almost one after the other, a few days apart.

First dream:

> *I am seven months pregnant when I dream that my baby comes out with his head on backward. My husband and I joke about it; we call him the devil baby. The doctor says, "Don't worry, we can fix it."*

Second dream:

> *I am still seven months pregnant when I have this next dream. I think it happened a week later. In my mind they somehow go together. In the dream I give birth to an angel, a winged child. I feel that my baby is one of the angels who has been called to earth at this time. It is a very mystical experience. After the baby arrives, the doctor feels the baby's back with his hands. He turns the baby around and notices big wings, long arched bloody wings, very realistic. The bloody veins scare me. The doctor tilts the baby to the side. When the baby is completely out, he opens his wings and takes a big breath. The baby has the bluest eyes you could imagine. When I*

look into those eyes, I get the feeling that I am
staring into piercing truth.

These two dreams are two sides of the same coin. In the first dream, the baby comes out with his head on backward, slightly reminiscent of *The Exorcist*. But the nonchalant, even humorous attitude of the parents and the assurance from the doctor that he can "fix it" show that the dream should be taken with perhaps more than one grain of salt.

This woman's psyche jumps from one extreme to the other. In the next dream the baby goes from being a devil to an angel. It is interesting to note that in this case the angel is not pristine or otherworldly, but possessed with scary bloody wings and blue eyes that can pierce you with their truth. The words *avenging angel* come to mind.

In both cases, the unconscious mind is playing with and stretching the woman's ideas and beliefs about her baby. Her psyche is also trying to reach a balance between perfectly evil and perfectly good. To integrate both sides in the mind of the dreamer, the psyche calms her fears with a humorous version of *The Exorcist* and relaxes her heavenly expectations with a bloody angel.

Labor dreams run the gamut from being realistic to esoteric. Whether they include an airplane ride, blessed keys, or fallen angels, labor dreams are above all a rehearsal process for the mother-to-be. In one way or another, the dream world is giving the pregnant woman the opportunity to see herself go through labor and delivery. Not only can a woman ask for the personal accounts of her relatives and friends, but she can ask her own unconscious to provide her with dream memories that will be of assistance to her during her own labor. Though not necessarily prophetic, dreams of labor can be illuminating and comforting. They can establish an inner connection the mother-to-be can rely on if things feel overwhelming and out of control during labor.

In general, dreams of the third trimester carry a great store of images and memories that the mother-to-be can avail herself of during her time of giving birth. The following exercises are based on the idea that the images in third-trimester dreams are suggestions from the unconscious, and are designed to be used during labor as a focusing tool for the mother-to-be.

EXERCISES

Anchoring the Animal

If you have a strong connection to a dream animal such as a whale or an elephant (as previously described in this chapter), then make up your mind that this animal will be your guardian, your helper, during your labor. Of course, it can be any animal you dreamed of that had a profound and positive impact on you. The reason it is better to choose a dream image rather than a random one from your waking life is because if your own unconscious chose it, then it is usually because this particular animal has special attributes that relate specifically to the essence of your being.

Here is how the exercise works:

- Practice your ability to summon the image of the animal into your mind.
- List the attributes of the animal: wise, patient, compassionate, ancient, whatever comes to you when you think of an elephant or a dolphin or whatever it is.
- Saturate your imagination with physical and emotional details.
- Get a beautiful photograph or a poster depicting the animal you have chosen.
- Make it real, make the animal your friend in your waking life as well as your nights.

The more you invest your energy into this dream image, the more available it will be to you during labor. You will be able to summon this animal and draw on its wisdom, its strength, its patience and ancient knowledge. It will be your friend, your guardian, your personal guide.

Practice this exercise as much as you can. I recommend doing the anchoring of the dream image just before going to sleep and just after you wake up. These transition times are very powerful as I have mentioned in previous chapters. The body is relaxed, the mind is open and receptive, and the imagination is clear.

Anchoring the Star

A dream of a movie star can provide the same kind of anchor as a dream of an animal, benefiting the woman who is giving birth. Besides the obvious differences, the star dreams have their own appeal. The energy they can generate, if used properly, can be very helpful to the woman during her labor.

- If the star is a man, make a list of his physical attributes. Is he a hunk? Is he strong? Is he masculine?
- Get in touch with your feelings about the star. Does he make you feel safe, protected, secure?
- Find out whether this dream image lifts your spirits and reassures you.
- Does the image of the star help you feel beautiful, like a whole woman?

If the rapport you establish with the dream image of the star makes you feel beautiful, safe, strengthened by his presence, then do not hesitate to use it in the same manner you would use any positive image.

- Let the star be an anchor for you during your labor. Your unconscious has chosen this particular star because of the qualities you believe he possesses.
- Allow these qualities to help you prepare yourself psychically and emotionally for the labor.
- Conjure up in your mind's eye not just the image of the star but the qualities he evokes in you.
- Do this until you can summon at will the feelings of safety, reassurance, wholeness, and whatever else this dream image inspires.
- Cultivate your awareness of the feelings that the star arouses in you. These feelings will serve you well during your birthing journey.

As with the previous exercise, rehearse your experience of these comforting feelings as much as possible, especially before sleep and after you first wake up, while still in bed.

• • •

When the dream image is a female star, allow yourself to identify with her qualities. Again your dreamlife has chosen this particular image because of the qualities you believe she possesses. Open yourself up to the image from your dream and let your imagination soar.

- List all the qualities you feel the star possesses: courage, wisdom, strength, beauty, equanimity, self-control, resilience, talent, charisma.
- Take each quality one at a time and allow yourself to merge with it. Explore what the resilience, self-control, or courage this star embodies would feel like for you.
- Practice owning each quality for a short period of time until it becomes second nature. Start small and keep expanding. You might find that you want to spend a lot of time feeling these feelings!
- Associate the picture of the star in your mind's eye with a particular quality you want to experience. You can even decide to have the star dress differently to match a specific feeling. Each outfit should conjure up a particular quality you want to feel. Make it fun. Be a "fashion designer" and a "feeling designer" all at the same time.
- Practice summoning a specific image of the star with its concomitant feeling. Practice in the morning before you get up and at night before you go to sleep. Practice any time you have a quiet moment. Enjoy feeling like a star, beautiful, competent, resilient—a winner.

Star-filled dreams are a way for the psyche to communicate with the mother-to-be. They offer examples of qualities and feelings the pregnant woman can anchor in her consciousness with these exercises and draw upon, like a reservoir, during labor.

Anchoring the Labor

With dreams of labor and delivery, you can use your own dream images as a model for the kind of labor you want to have, physically and emotionally. Here is how it works:

- First, select an image from a labor dream that you feel strongly about. It should be memorable, containing specific qualities related to the labor that felt vivid and right for you. It could be that you experienced a short labor or that you felt a great connection with your unborn child during the whole process. It could be that you had very little pain or that the joy of seeing your child for the first time was the most overwhelming thing on your mind.
- Once you have selected an image, begin to rehearse it in your mind until it becomes real for you, as real as it was in the dream.
- Use your imagination to fill the image with whatever sensations you think should be present. What are the contractions like? Are you hot, damp, tired? What does the room look like, smell like? Who is in the room with you?
- Create as complete an image as you are able. Draw a picture if that helps you.
- Let the image from the labor dream sink into your mind until it becomes as familiar as a memory.

- Play a game with yourself. See how many times a day you can bring up the memory you made up with the help of your dream image.
- The closer you are to your due date, the more you should practice.

If you had a dream with a female movie star, you might want to use it during the most intense or painful part of your labor in the couvade fashion. Simply tell yourself that during the most intense parts of the labor, Meryl Streep (or whoever it is for you) will go through the symptoms of the labor on your behalf and that you will not feel any pain. Repeat this sentence to yourself during transition times before sleep and after you wake up or during any quiet time. You can use it as a mantra, a silent phrase you say to yourself during a moment of relaxation. Make it a meditation.

Do this only if you feel comfortable with the idea. It is a very powerful process that can really help alleviate your pain temporarily, just like an epidural, but in this case you are the one creating your own painkiller with your imagination. The painkiller is the movie star from your own dream.

With any of the anchoring exercises, be sure that the image you choose is one that not only has great emotional resonance with your being, but also makes you feel supported, powerful, loved, and calm. Most of all, choose an image that makes you feel relaxed and comfortable, one that you can work with over and over again without getting bored. In fact the more you play with the image and meditate on it, the more enjoyment you will receive.

Be sure that the dream image you have picked as an anchor for your labor has the qualities you require to carry you through this decisive time. Don't wait until you are in the middle of a gigantic contraction to figure out whether your anchor is working for you or not. Take the time to examine and test it. Imagine that you are in the middle of labor. How do you think this anchor will perform under pressure? Will it be easy for you to hold its picture in your mind's eye? Will its qualities or traits really be nourishing for you? Will it help you in the exact manner that you need it to? Be thorough. Your level of comfort and your ability to relax and trust in between the contractions may depend on it.

PART II

❧

Premonitory Dreams and Other Mystical Experiences

❧

Premonitory or psychic dreams can occur at different times during a woman's life, but during the time of her pregnancy this kind of phenomenon tends to occur most frequently. Some people say that it is because a pregnant woman is in peak physical health that she becomes a clear channel for psychic perceptions. (Mothers-to-be tend to give up any habits that might be detrimental to the healthy growth of their baby such as smoking, drinking alcohol, or even eating spicy and fried foods.) Other people claim that it is all hormonal, that it is the internal tempest in a woman's body that causes her to have visions and premonitions. And there are other studies that claim that a pregnant woman experiences psychic dreams because at this time in her life she tends to be more quiet and contemplative than ever before, able to pay attention to the subtle currents in her psyche that would otherwise be left unexplored.

Whatever it is, this phenomenon is common enough among pregnant women to warrant further study. Consequently, this part of the book will be dedicated to the types of psychic dreams that occur most frequently during pregnancy and the circumstances that surround them.

From the interviews I have collected, it has become apparent that most psychic dreams of pregnant women give insights into the sex of the child. These psychic dreams usually occur in the second trimester, at a time when the mother begins to bond with her unborn baby. But this time frame is not written in stone. Psychic dreams are not bound by time and space, and there are examples of this category of dreams happening days or even weeks before the woman becomes pregnant. In such dreams, the baby's distinct personality imposes itself upon the mother's psyche from an invisible plane of existence.

In 90 percent of the cases the dreams turn out to be a correct assessment of the child's sex and personality. The mistake in gender usually comes from a misinterpretation of the dream, not the dream itself.

There are also purely psychic dreams that do not immediately relate to the pregnancy. These dreams can range from a straightforward premonition all the way to an awe-inspiring mystical experience, rich in soulful gifts. These dreams tend to make an indelible impression on the mother-to-be and usually resurface during traumatic events, such as labor, when emotional or psychological support is needed. So although these dreams do not at first seem to have an obvious connection to the pregnancy, they can take an unexpected yet significant place during the birthing process.

CHAPTER FOUR

Dreams of the Baby's Sex

During the second trimester a woman's awareness that a human being is growing in her womb can foster great excitement about the sex of the baby. If the mother-to-be has issues regarding women or men that have not yet been resolved—such as "men are violent" or "women are bossy"—then dreams about the sex of the baby could flourish around that time. These dreams can be an opportunity for the mother-to-be to take a good look at her beliefs about men and women and come to some resolution or acceptance about the matter.

So even if all you are interested in is the sex of your baby, premonition dreams have other valuable components. Not only do they answer questions concerning the gender of your child, such dreams also create an opening for healing to take place on a psychological and emotional level. They enhance the contact between the mother and the child, creating a pathway through which vital information may be passed.

Lucy is the mother of three boys, and psychic dreams relating to the gender of her baby were a normal second-trimester occurrence during each of her pregnancies. Because the sex of the baby was integrated into her dreams, Lucy did not make anything of it until the doctor told her she was having a boy and she remembered that she had already dreamed about it. As she said to me in our interview, "It was amazing to realize that part of me already knew my baby was a boy." The full impact of the dream came only with the actual birth of her baby when she saw that he looked exactly like he had in the dream.

Lucy's third pregnancy was a little different. Both she and her husband did not want to know the sex of the baby because they were hoping that after the birth of two boys they would have a girl. Much to her surprise, during the pregnancy with her third child, Lucy had a dream that revealed to her that her final offspring would indeed also be of the male gender. The comfort and acceptance emanating from the dream helped Lucy accept the gift of her third child even though it was not a girl. The next two dreams are from her first and third pregnancies.

> In the dream, I am in a hospital room. I have just given birth to my baby. It is very clear that he is a boy. I think to myself that my baby reminds me of an ex-boyfriend of mine, my first love who was from South America. I marvel at

the baby's size. He is stocky and quite strong looking, a little football player in the making. My husband and I are getting him dressed to go home from the hospital. He has a lot of curly hair and he is rather dark. His feet are so large that I put toddler-size sandals on him to go home.

Lucy explained to me afterward that when her son was born she remembered this dream because he looked identical to what she had seen while sleeping—dark-skinned and chunky. Since both Lucy and her husband were fair-skinned, it was an odd vision to have. She felt strangely relieved when the baby turned blond a few weeks later.

Somehow, her baby's dark curly hair brought up a lot of feelings for her about an ex-boyfriend, a fellow who would pop up in her dreams at odd times in her life. The psychic dream not only revealed the sex of her baby, but also gave her the opportunity to look at some of the lingering beliefs she had about men, triggered by the resemblance of her baby to her ex-boyfriend. Though Lucy had been madly in love with this man, it had proved to be a very dysfunctional and abusive relationship. Because of this, Lucy started to see men as a dangerous and untrustworthy breed. When her baby turned out to look just like the type of men she shunned in her waking life, it forced her to deal with the anger and resentment she still held toward her ex-lover.

This psychic dream was incredibly accurate not only in its depiction of what the baby would look like when it was first born, but also in how it reminded Lucy of her ex-boyfriend. Thanks to the dream, Lucy was able to eradicate the subconscious beliefs that might have negatively impacted the way she raised her baby boy. She embarked on a healing path because she did not want her maternal love to be tainted by the negative feelings her passionate and painful history with that man had generated.

In the psychic dream about her third baby, the feelings that surrounded the dream were very evocative. Lucy's unconscious displayed a very delicate and private emotional tone that was wonderfully expressed by the symbology of the dream. Lucy explained to me that she and her husband did not want to know the sex of the baby, but that she assumed she would have a dream about it simply because it had happened for both of her previous pregnancies. She was not too surprised when it happened six months into the pregnancy. What was fascinating to her was the accuracy of the feelings she was having in the dream. It was as if the dream knew better than she did what her feelings were. The dream really helped her that way. She was able to deal with her emotional state much more easily once the dream brought it to her conscious awareness.

> *I am at a make-believe park. My other two boys are not with me. I am holding my precious new baby underneath the swing set. People, family and friends, are all coming up to me and asking if it's a boy or a girl. I tell them it is a boy. I get a lot of sympathy from everyone. They are all disappointed that it is a boy, and they leave me under the swing set. I feel very quiet and protective of my baby, relieved that they are not going to fuss and make a huge deal out of it, which they would have if it was a girl. No pink dresses*

*and no pink parties, just me and my baby. I am
filled with love for my baby. I don't want anybody around. I wake up knowing that I just had
a psychic dream about the sex of my baby.*

In this touching dream, Lucy's feelings about having
a boy are revealed. There is a sense that she must protect
the baby from everyone. She is almost hiding under the
swing set. Lucy is alone with her baby. They are in a very
private world with no one else; not even her other children are there to disturb them. In the dream, she is glad
that the people go away when they find out it is not the
much anticipated girl. The mother much prefers the
calm of their isolated bliss to the pink fuss that would
have occurred with the birth of a girl. There is a distinct
overall feeling of contentment, acceptance, and even
satisfaction about the outcome of the pregnancy, which
shows a mother's love for her baby, regardless of its sex.

Psychic dreams about the sex of the baby can involve
other distinct elements besides holding significance
about our beliefs toward men and women. In some cases
the woman will feel the dream as a nudge from the
baby, showing the mother-to-be that she needs to make
space for its arrival. This often contributes to a mother's
urgent desire for a new home, a more comfortable nest
for herself and her expanding family.

Holly's dream convinced her that she would have a
girl, but it was only after a closer examination that she
acknowledged the ensuing role the dream had played in
her decision to move to a new house at the end of her
second trimester. She found herself knee-deep in boxes
right until the last minute, which is not what she
expected at all.

I am in the bedroom with my husband watching television when I realize that I am watching this very clear picture of myself trying to stop my baby girl from falling off the bookshelf. There is no room to turn. Our place is clearly too small. And my little girl is very upset about it. She is kicking and screaming as if she wanted me to make space for her. I wake up knowing that I am going to have a little girl.

Soon after she had this dream, Holly started to feel very claustrophobic in their little one-bedroom apartment. She told her husband that they needed more space. She wanted the baby to feel welcome. She wanted a little garden. Upon examining the dream again, she realized that there was more to it than her premonition about having a baby girl. She began to wonder if her resoluteness about moving in the middle of her pregnancy had not been instigated by the baby herself, already imposing her own will on the world. In the dream, the baby girl had been very clear about her displeasure with the present situation and her demands for more space. This thought struck a deep chord in Holly, as if her baby was controlling her through her dreams. The mother-to-be was in awe of this force of Nature who demanded to have her needs met from the other side. It became clear to Holly that she was responding to greater needs than her own. Her pregnancy took on a more mystical aura from that moment on, as she became aware of the mysterious ramifications of carrying this little bundle in her womb.

Some psychic dreams about the baby's sex can be misinterpreted because of other important elements. In this case the dreamer is literally sidetracked by certain symbols or characters in the dreams that have their own agenda and messages to impart. Susan's dream is such an example. There are two children in her dream, and Susan makes the assumption that the older, more expressive one is the baby she is going to have, rather than the quiet younger one. She does not realize that the older child might have an altogether different function in her dream.

> *In the dream, I am in the car, driving with a four-year-old redheaded little girl. She has a very strong presence, telling me where to go and what to do. I am fascinated with this determined little redhead. She is quite a character with a very strong will. She seems to know exactly what to do, and when, even if she is not the one actually doing the driving. She is definitely in charge. The girl's presence is so overwhelming in fact that I barely notice the quiet little boy strapped in a baby chair in the backseat. I wake up thinking that I am going to have a little girl and that she will be very strong-willed.*

Susan was shocked when she had a quiet and adorable little boy instead of the redheaded girl she expected. But when she remembered the dream, she realized that she had completely dismissed the fact that the little boy was in fact present in the dream, sitting in the backseat with the same quiet sweet presence her baby had in real life. The problem, or the mistake Susan had made in interpreting her dream, was that the redhead had such a striking personality and presence that she overshadowed the baby boy.

Who was this strong-willed little girl?

Upon further examination, Susan felt a very strong tie to her. Also, the little girl was not just strong-willed, but held a lot of wisdom, knowing exactly where to go and what to do, guiding the mother and child safely, with a little extra force. It was almost a case of child knows best. But this was no ordinary child. It was a dream child and an old soul, according to Susan. This redhead relied on her instincts and trusted them perfectly. She was intuitive and spoke with a matter-of-fact attitude. She knew when she was on the right track and what to do to get back on it. She was Susan's perfect instinctual self, the being she was before the emotional and psychological wounds of her own childhood had left their indelible mark, separating her from that powerful and wise child. Becoming pregnant was an avenue for Susan to heal not only that instinctual self, but literally to put it back in charge. Susan's pregnancy instigated a resurrection of all her instincts that might have been buried with the painful past or even forgotten. This vital guiding force was perfectly embodied in the dream by the little redheaded girl.

Psychic dreams about the sex of your child are filled with gifts just like any other dreams. They can show you the beliefs you harbor about men and women. They can guide you to new emotional and psychological depths. They can provide a safe haven for delicate feelings and show you the way back to your instinctual self. And though the idea of even having a psychic dream might be bothersome to you, do not let your preconceptions stand in the way of meeting that little redhead who has been waiting so long for you to let her speak up and guide you and your baby to safety.

EXERCISES

The Sex of the Baby

If you wake up from a psychic dream about the sex of your baby, do not immediately try to analyze it or figure out whether it is really a premonition. Be still and allow the dream to wash through your consciousness until the most important elements or symbols from the dream rise to the surface and stay with you. Then ask yourself the following questions:

- Where is the dream taking place? Are the surroundings familiar?
- What does the baby look like?
- How does the sex of the baby affect me?
- Do I feel good about the fact that I might have a boy/girl?
- Does the thought of having a girl/boy worry or frighten me? Why?
- Where do these feelings come from?

Whether the dream turns out to be a real premonition or not does not matter. What is important is that you had a dream about the sex of your baby. Examining the feelings surrounding the dream might help you establish a healthy relationship with your baby right from the start.

If it is crucial to your peace of mind to find out the sex of your baby, you might want to try this next exercise (of course, you can also get accurate information from an amniocentesis or ultrasound). It is a simplified method of autosuggestion or a mild form of self-hypnosis that is done right before sleep. If you need more information, you can refer to other exercises in Parts II and III.

Before Going to Sleep

When you are already in bed with the lights out, take three relaxing breaths. Then hold your breath in to a count of ten if you can, then release it like a pressure valve exploding. After these three breaths, bring your breath back to a calm, quiet hum as if you were already asleep. When you feel yourself drifting into sleep, repeat the following three statements:

1. Tonight I will have a psychic dream about the sex of my baby.
2. When I wake up I will remember my dream.
3. I will know with absolute certainty the sex of my child.

Repeat these three statements over and over like a mantra. Do not worry if you fall asleep in the middle of it. Your unconscious will continue the work for you.

After You Wake Up

Be still. Let the dream images float up to the surface of your mind. Do not judge what you remember. Be convinced that there is an answer, maybe not the one you want, but there is some form of a response to your question. If the dream is not immediately clear, ask the following questions:

• Is there a symbol in the dream that reminds me of a boy/girl?
• Is there something I am not seeing or understanding?
• What is obvious?
• What is absent?
• If I really trusted the dream, what would it be telling me?

This last question is the key. Do not second-guess yourself. Trust your unconscious and your instincts as a mother-to-be. As one of the women I interviewed said, "I have never felt so intuitive in my life; my dreams have never been so vivid nor so prophetic."

Whether you have premonitions about the sex of your baby, or call these types of dreams forth with the power of your mind, by the end of the second trimester you have formed the most intimate connection with another human being you will ever have. The very nature of this connection is profoundly intuitive. How could it not be when you are carrying a human being inside your own womb, feeding him/her with your body, your blood beating two hearts? The premonitory dreams are not an extraordinary event, but should be considered a natural occurrence, self-evident, and mysteriously ordinary, like life.

CHAPTER FIVE

Beyond Time and Space

Psychic dreams about the sex of the baby can take on an added mystery when they step across the boundaries of time and space. These dreams tend to leave an indelible impression on the dreamer: Their luminous quality makes them memorable.

These dreams are always very vivid. They contain powerful symbols and crisp colors, whether they take place outdoors, in a landscape-type setting, or indoors in a kitchen or a bedroom. Usually, it is not only the sex of the child that is revealed in these psychic dreams, but some other special quality about the future personality of the baby or even the circumstances of the birth.

Sometimes a pregnant woman in her second trimester will be given the gift of seeing what her child will look and act like years into the future. These dreams are not easily dismissed or set aside even by the most skeptical among us. When life finally catches up with these nighttime premonitions, months or years from now, it often affects the dreamer like déjà vu, with a great surge of energy that knowing something from deep within, before it ever happened, can provide.

Psychic dreams, even when they are filled with meaningful information, are never ominous. They are akin to taking fresh mountain air into your lungs after spending an inordinate amount of time breathing smog. They open your conscious mind to a wider range of experiences, a store of wisdom you did not even know you had, an ancient knowledge that your ancestors used as a matter of course. During your pregnancy you have the possibility and the opportunity of becoming your own oracle (or augur as the Romans called it) through your personal nightly stories. The connection between you and your baby can advance until you are on the same psychic wavelength, able to communicate back and forth from soul to soul.

A year and a half before she became pregnant, Maddix had a dream about a child that she came to see as a positive symbol of her future with the man she was in love with. This dream affected her deeply. For her it was an affirmation that she was indeed in a relationship with the right person. It made sense to Maddix to have a dream about a baby who looked a lot like her boyfriend at the time, if she was meant to continue her involvement with this man. They had been at an important juncture in their relationship, and for Maddix the dream proved to be an affirmation and a confirmation that their relationship was worth the effort and that it was time for them to move to the next level of commitment. A standard explanation of the dream was that the baby was an expression of their love, of what was being born between the two of them. The truth is that this was not only a symbolic dream, but a real psychic dream about the future child Maddix would have with her partner and what he would look like as a toddler.

> *I am walking on the beach. The sun is shining on the water like a million stars. The air is warm and there is a breeze. Everything is shimmering, gleaming. I have short hair in the dream and I am dressed in white. I am with a boy who is also dressed in white. The boy is about one year old, a toddler. He has golden hair like my boyfriend. We are drawing shapes together in the sand with our feet. I feel as if I have been doing this for-ever. There is no sense of time at all. It is hap-pening now. I know this is my child.*

When Maddix woke up, she felt certain that the child she saw in her dream would one day be her real son. The dream gave her confidence that she was with the right man and that he would indeed be the father. It was an extremely positive dream for her that Maddix trusted without being able to explain why. She knew wholeheartedly that her unconscious was signaling to her that it was time to start preparing herself for a future baby. Consequently, she began to pay more attention to her body and took better care of herself. She wanted to make her body ready to receive her future child in as healthy a manner as possible.

Looking back on the dream—as the current mother of a baby boy with hair the color of honey wheat—it was easy for Maddix to see how psychic and reassuring her dream was. It prompted her to conceive a child and prepared her for the trials of pregnancy. Her dream had been both a meaningful, comforting symbol as well as an omen for the birth of her baby boy. Her instinctual self received the dream as a gift and was able to use it to guide her into the rich frontiers of motherhood.

Psychic dreams of future children often take place in similar settings of sandy beaches and calm seas, with gleaming sparkles of reflected sunlight. The limitless oceanic landscape, the white sand, the waves are all symbolic of the feminine principle of life. Between land and water, on the wet sandy shore, the invisible and visible can meet and new life can be born. Time and space become irrelevant. The truth is revealed freely. A mother can play with her future offspring. Together they can draw circles in the sand with their feet, the circles of life, without beginning and without end.

Another mother-to-be had a similarly arresting dream just before a planned move to Hawaii during the second trimester of her pregnancy. The symbology of the dream is extremely vivid. The messages that are given are psychic in nature and speak to the mother-to-be with startling accuracy.

> *I am dreaming that I am already in Maui, an island of Hawaii, where we are moving to in real life. I am climbing this mountain, which turns out to be a volcano. In Hawai the tallest peak is actually a volcano called Haleakala Crater. I think this is the mountain I am climbing in my dream. I finally get to the top and I look into the*

crater. There I see a beautiful golden-haired woman with two fetuses at her feet. The fetuses turn into a boy and a girl. They are lying there in the crater. I hear a voice. I am not sure if it is the golden-haired woman speaking or not, but nonetheless the voice is talking to me. It is saying that these are my children and that they will be born under the sign of Gemini.

When the mother-to-be found out a few months later that she was going to have fraternal twins and that they would be born under the astrological sign of Gemini, she could not help but realize how portentous and accurate her dream had been.

She had first taken the dream as a good omen for the projected move to Hawaii. When she found out about the exact nature of her pregnancy, she had to take a closer look at this memorable dream.

A volcano, with its fire coming straight from the center of the earth, is a powerful metaphor for the life force that is activated during pregnancy and birth. The blonde woman sitting in the crater itself is another wonderful expression of the feminine power that women connect with once they conceive a child. This character is also a symbol of the woman's higher self or, in Jungian terminology, what analysts call the anima. She is the one who knows things beyond time and space, the oracle aspect of a woman's inner nature, the intuitive self, the soul. She presents the mother-to-be with the news about her future children. She makes her declaration in a very particular setting, right near the fiery cauldron of the volcano, which is symbolic of the womb of the earth, a perfect metaphor for the creative force that women can generate. The blonde woman brings clear and precise information about the exact nature of the children, their sex and astrological sign.

There is something innately mystical in the dream and the information it is bringing forth. This woman had always instinctively honored the wisdom available in her night stories, but she was overwhelmed by the psychic strength her dreams took on during her pregnancy. Like others in her condition, she had the genuine sense that her intuition was at an all-time high during her entire pregnancy and that her dreams reflected this heightened sensitivity in their content as well as their luminous quality. Never before in her life had she felt so in tune with her creative energy. Never before had she known so clearly that she was personally connected to the mystery of life.

Nancy is another mother-to-be who used the word *luminous* to describe a dream she had at the end of her second trimester. Psychic dreams were not a regular part of her life, and yet when she had this particular dream, she knew instinctively that it expressed something that down the road would manifest itself in her daily reality. There was something so truthful and ordinary about the dream that it took on the atmosphere of a genuine experience of time travel. In fact, it took about seven years for Nancy to verify the authenticity of her dream. The truth is, this mother-to-be could never forget the dream because she knew in her heart of hearts that it was real.

In the dream, I am in our new house. We had actually just moved in the month before. I am standing in the kitchen of our new house, looking at a seven- or eight-year-old in school uniform. She is a tall, slender dark-haired little girl, who looks awfully like my Native American husband. I can't take my eyes off of her. I am trying to talk to her but she doesn't listen or, rather, she doesn't think I know what I am talking about. She is very strong-willed. I tell her that I don't like her hitchhiking home from school. She is annoyed with me. It is very clear that she does not like me telling her what to do. She thinks I am too fearful. She says to me, "Mommy, it's fine," in that exasperated little-girl tone. I know I am not getting through to her, so I say, "You are hard-headed just like your mother." I wake up.

Nancy knew right away that the girl she had seen in her dream was her own daughter as she would be at the age of seven. It worried her a little to have such a strong-willed daughter until she remembered that in the dream, she herself had said that the little girl was hard-headed just like her mother. So the dream, besides showing her a vivid picture of the future personality, sex, and appearance of her child, was also a hint for herself. It was an opportunity for her to look at her own stubbornness and determine for herself whether or not it served her in her daily life.

Nancy did not know the sex of her child at the time she had this dream. When she found out she was having a daughter, it was a confirmation that she had indeed had a psychic dream, not only about the sex of the child but also about her personality and her looks.

Standing with her daughter in their home seven years later, Nancy can now reflect on this extraordinary dream and embrace its full impact. Her daughter is that very same slender, tall, dark-haired little girl who was first presented to her in this psychic dream years earlier. Nancy is grateful that her daughter is not quite as petulant as she was in the dream. But then again, the dream showed her what could be, the possibilities, and her own maturing process as a woman and a mother has no doubt affected the character of their relationship.

Superimposing the images from the dream over the reality as it presents itself now, one beholds an almost perfect match, which transcends our definitions of reality. Time and space become blurred, and a more cosmic view of the world emerges, not so linear, not so flat, a world to which Nancy was intimately connected during her pregnancy.

The intuitive dialogue a woman has with life is never more apparent than during her pregnancy. Her ability to dream the future, to see clearly in her night visions what her baby will not only look like, but also his/her personality, is a testimony to the fact that human relationships are not limited by time or space and that they can occur on separate planes of existence. We are only limited in our perception of what is real by our beliefs. Bringing forth a brand-new human being can be a life-changing experience in more ways than one. It can expand our beliefs about the very meaning of life. It can allow us to break down seemingly impenetrable boundaries between the conscious and unconscious mind. It can help us face hidden dimensions of our character and integrate them into a more harmonious whole.

The treasures hidden in psychic dreams often take years to come to fruition. Invariably they prove to be an asset in the person's life, a discovery or an insight into their own character, as well as offering valuable clues into the relationship they have established with their child.

Having numerous psychic dreams is a natural occurrence among pregnant women. Their amazing capacity to have such dreams does not make it any less ordinary. This is no paranormal phenomenon. It is precisely what happens when you accept within your body and your soul the mysterious beauty of life.

EXERCISE

Psychic Meditation

Because you already have an enhanced intuitive ability during pregnancy, this is the best time in your life to develop your psychic perceptions.

• Make some time for yourself, half an hour or more if you can. Begin with inhaling deeply and holding your breath for a count of ten. Then breathe out completely. Do this three times as in the previous exercises. Allow a natural sense of letting go, like a soothing touch, to come over you with the out breath. Pay attention to that feeling of surrender and relaxation. It is the key. The depth of your letting go is a mirror of your ability to give up the habitual thought processes from your daily life.

• You can do this exercise alone or you can invite your partner to join you. If you can synchronize your breathing, the energy you will both feel will be much stronger and carry you further than you would go on your own. It will be easier to break down the barriers of your mind-set, provided there is a concerted effort on both sides.

• Once you have completed the three breaths of letting go, begin the quiet breath. This method of breathing, as I have said earlier, is akin to the breath of sleep. The spirit can rest lightly in the body with such a breath. Nothing is forced or labored. It is effortless, indiscernible. It allows the heart rate to slow down and the mind to calm down. Have you noticed how the more you think, the quicker your breathing becomes and the faster your heart beats? The reverse is also true: The softer the breathing, the more restful the heart, the calmer the mind.

• Begin to concentrate on the space between your eyebrows, directly above the bridge of the nose. This space between the eyebrows is called the third eye in many Eastern religions. You can even imagine a vertical eye on that spot if it helps you. I often put my middle finger on my forehead for a brief moment just to connect with that spot. It helps me shift my attention to less petty, more soulful concerns.

• Close your eyes if you have not done so already and turn them up toward that space between your eyebrows. Do not worry if this is hard to do. It does not have to be done perfectly. Feel your breath going into that space, bringing it to life softly, powerfully.

• Visualize a light shining in your third eye. It could be a bright flame, unless the idea of a star or the sun inspires you more. Whatever you decide, make it bright and strong. Give it a specific hue. It should be a color that moves you. For some, blue is peaceful; for others green is always a reminder of the richness of nature. Whether red or pink, white or yellow, pick a color for the flame that is easy for you to imagine and comfortable to stare into.

• Once the colored flame is clear in your mind's eye, let it expand and fill your awareness like a vast ocean. With each breath, let the flame spill out even more and envelop everything around you.

• Imagine that it reaches up into the sky, past the atmosphere of our planet, fills out our solar system, and at the speed of light, goes right through the entire Milky Way and into the cosmic darkness, shedding its lovely light. Allow into your mind the idea that as your light expands beyond the reaches of human possibilities, your consciousness is similarly stretched.

• Repeat to yourself until it rings absolutely true:
  • I am connected to the whole universe.
  • I am here and I am on the other side of space and time.
  • The past and the future are an open book in the eternal now of my life.
  • My consciousness is infinite.
  • I am one with the consciousness of the universe.
  • I live in the world of infinite possibilities. If you are a scientist by inclination or by profession, you can change the words slightly and say instead:
  • I live in the world of infinite probabilities.
  • Psychic moments are a natural part of my life.
• You can choose one of the above sentences to work

with on a regular basis or you can make up your own. One of my personal favorites is: The past and the future are an open book in the eternal now of my life. The image of this book is so right for me that the light in my third eye can become like a laser pointing to and illuminating the great book of life in the timeless sky. My second favorite sentence is: Psychic moments are a natural part of my life.

• Once you have become accustomed to the idea of having a third eye, use it to focus on specific problems in your life you do not have an obvious solution for. In other words, instead of figuring things out logically, try locating with your third eye a solution from your higher self. To do this, simply hold the problem in the light of your third eye until it is bathing in the light. Surrender all preconceived notions of what and how your problem should work out. Trust that your psychic mind will come up with the best possible scenario. If an answer does not reach you immediately, expect to get it while you are busy doing something else or in your dreamtime.

• You can use this technique with a new person, a potential business partner or lover. Hold them in the light of your third eye and see what is revealed.

• If you do this exercise on a regular basis, you will develop your psychic abilities quickly. You will start seeing things not only with your eyes or your mind, but with an expanded consciousness that does not recognize the human limitations of space and time.

• Finally, you can focus the light of your third eye on your potential or future baby. You can imagine a link being established between your flame and his/hers and thus begin a psychic dialogue even before you become pregnant.

This psychic meditation is a tool to expand your consciousness beyond its current limitations. Its purpose will be defeated if you approach it with a closed, skeptical mind and negative ideas about what it means to be psychic. I hope I have made it clear that being psychic is a natural expression of the mind. In most of us it lies dormant, but at the time of pregnancy, the psychic potential of women blossoms in the wake of the new life being created within.

If you choose to cultivate this potential at this time, it will remain with you long after your pregnancy has reached its completion and you have given birth. Your natural intuition will be enhanced and your daily life will provide you with countless opportunities to test your psychic potential, especially with your newborn baby.

Like the milk from your breasts that pours forth when the baby cries with hunger, your psychic line to your baby will be tugged upon by the unconditional bond of love established between the two of you before birth.

CHAPTER SIX

Purely Psychic Dreams

The psychic content of dreams by pregnant women is not limited to the subject of babies and motherhood. It can sometimes contain psychic information about friends or relatives and their lives, and have no direct relation to the dreamer, her pregnancy, or the sex of the baby. These types of dreams are what I call purely psychic dreams, and women in their second trimester seem more available to this type of information than at any other time in their life. The natural enhancement of their psychic abilities, whether hormonal or otherwise, makes women a greater channel for such timeless information.

One particular woman had a series of dreams on the cusp between her second and third trimester about a friend's dog. This would not have been extremely noteworthy except that the series of dreams depicted the dog getting lost and later revealed the circumstances in which it was eventually found. The dreams were so accurate and precise that their premonitory quality could not be denied. Indeed, they turned out to be thoroughly exact in their description. It was as if this woman's unconscious knew things she did not know consciously but was nevertheless connected to on a subliminal level. She was not too surprised because she had felt "more intuitive than I ever have in my life" from the beginning of her pregnancy and even in the months preceding her becoming pregnant.

In my first dream, Jezebel, who is Beatrice's dog, has been lost for several days. I am sitting outside my store in the parking lot with a very handsome hairdresser. He does not have time to give me a haircut. I know that Jezebel is coming back.

In the second dream a few days later, I dream again that Beatrice's dog is coming back to her. This time there is an old woman who is crying her heart out because she has to bring the dog back. She brings her to the store. Jezebel, the dog, badly needs a bath.

In the third dream, I am again sitting outside my store in the parking lot on a beach chair. Again I want to get a haircut from the very handsome hairdresser, but he does not have time. Then Jezebel, the dog, shows up. The dog keeps saying, "Mama, Mama," in the dream, just like

a baby would. Beatrice is with me this time. She
picks up her dog. She is so happy; she almost
cannot believe she found her little Jezebel.

After missing for two weeks, Jezebel came back. Reality mirrored the dream world as the dog was brought in by an old woman who was crying at the thought of giving up Jezebel, who, by the way, was in dire need of a bath.

The realism of the dream makes its extraneous elements stand out even more. For instance, there is the setting of the dream with the handsome hairdresser and the beach chair, and of course the way the dog cries out, "Mama, Mama." These symbols are intertwined with the premonitory message of the dream in a way that is particularly meaningful to the woman dreaming. Even in a purely psychic dream such as this one, the personality and the concerns of the dreamer are made manifest in the story.

The setting of the dream juxtaposes the practicality of a parking lot with the relaxed feeling one can associate with a beach chair. Sensuality is added to the mix with the character of the handsome hairdresser who does not have time to cut hair. This interesting detail of the handsome man refusing to cut the woman's hair illustrates how the woman's sexual energy is needed not for her own gratification but for the family she is creating.

The dog itself is a very powerful symbol, which deserves to be explored apart from its role in the premonitory aspect of the dream. In most cultures, the dog is seen as a faithful, loyal friend of human beings. A dog is someone who stays, or if lost, always endeavors to return to its master. One thinks of stories like *Lassie* and of the sled dogs of Alaska. A dog is often associated with family and hearth, and most people who own a dog consider it to be a bona fide member of the family.

In the dream, the dog is returned after being missing for two weeks. This speaks of the innate loyalty of the animal. However, there are many more meanings to the symbol of dog. Dog is also the fierce protector of not only the family but also of babies and the guardian of treasures in the underworld, the dream world.

This psychic dream is particularly interesting because of the central image of the dog. However true and realistic the story of the dream is, the dog is also a dream image that has a specific resonance for the dreamer, a resonance of friendship and loyalty and the protection of a family. Because of all this imagery associated with the dog symbol, such a dream, psychic or not, is very appropriate for a pregnant woman.

What makes this dream even more clearly relevant to the pregnancy is the fact that the dog repeats "Mama" twice when she is found. This speaks to the wild animal part of the woman, the "Jezebel" who rebelled against being tamed but who finally comes home, a little dirty, in need of a bath, accepting the life of family and the role of mother.

Even a dream such as this, a purely psychic dream, is not wasted on the dreamer. It is full of juicy bits of information about the state of mind of the woman, how she sees her transition from being her own person, sexually free, to a mother. For many women, with their first baby comes the realization, often for the first time, that "this is it, for real. I am now a responsible person, with a sacred commitment to another human being." It can often be a difficult transition, especially in our day and age when career and independence are valued so highly, and even psychic dreams like this can provide valuable tools for a transformative experience such as pregnancy and the birth of a child.

Psychic dreams can prove to be very exciting when they become realized. And as I have mentioned above, the unconscious does not waste a good dream on premonition alone. Everything that can be useful to the psychological development and emotional well-being of the dreamer is used.

This next dream has the same appearance of a purely psychic dream and yet functions very well as information for the pregnant woman. The dream itself is very simple and Deborah would not have conceived of it as a psychic dream if it had not come true the very next day. The dream happened toward the end of her second trimester.

> *It's a really pretty day, sunny, warm, not windy. I decide to go for a swim in the ocean in a special cove, which is quite private. I feel very hermitlike these days. I know I'll be okay. The waves are calm, and the area is protected from the bigger surf. I slowly go into the water. I am beginning to feel like a whale. I can't bear to think what it will be like a couple of months from now. The dream is so vivid. I'm thinking and feeling exactly the way I would if I was awake, doing the same thing. I start swimming, and all of a sudden I see a big animal coming to meet me. I don't panic even though it's so huge because it has a furlike coat. I recognize that it is a seal. It's a great big seal. It swims with me for*

a while. It makes me feel wonderful. The seal is not afraid of me either. There is a real communion between us, like she, the seal—I'm pretty sure it's a female—knows that I'm pregnant. I feel very privileged. When she leaves I go back to the beach and leave almost immediately. It's as if I came to the beach strictly to have this encounter. It's as if I was getting the seal of approval from Nature.

I have underlined the words *seal of approval* because they illustrate so plainly how the dream language often works in puns. Here the metaphor of the seal is used as a pun to show that the pregnant woman is in sync with life and her own nature. The seal is literally the "seal of approval."

The fact that Deborah decided to go swimming the next day and had to go alone because the friend she had invited to come with her canceled at the last minute, and the fact that she did end up swimming with a seal, just like in her dream—all of this does not take away from the dream standing on its own merit. It made the real encounter more meaningful. It was as if the dream was set up to help Deborah take notice, so that she would get the full benefit of the meeting when it happened the following day.

Many details of the dream are so luminous that the whole story takes on a mythical quality. Seals themselves have a very rich history of symbolism. Many traditions from Celtic to Native American have imbued seals with magical properties. Seals of the old tales could take off their skin and turn into beautiful maidens that men wanted to capture for their own. The energy of the seal is very loving, protective, and also very playful. They feed and play in the ocean, but choose to return to the earth for rest and relaxation as well as mating and giving birth.

You notice that in the dream the main reason our dreamer does not panic at the sight of this enormous animal is because of its coat. She recognizes that the seal is a mammal. There is an instinctual connection between the two, woman and seal, a similar energy, a recognition of the feminine power of life, which is both strong and playful.

This dream image would be perfect to use during labor as an ally. The seal would be a great companion for Deborah on her birthing journey if she chooses. The psychic quality of the dream followed by the live per- formance makes it a potentially very strong memory. The qualities of the seal, such as its strength, endurance, and even more important, its playfulness and trust, are precisely the kind of characteristics that make it the perfect anchor for labor. It is an image Deb- orah can go back to again and again to help remind her what this is all about: the joy, the ecstasy of bringing your own child into the world, and a glimpse at the eternal through the unconditional love painted a mil- lion times as the Madonna and Child.

Psychic dreams are rich in interpretation for friends and family around you as well as for yourself. The more informed people who are close to you are about what you are going through, the more they can be there for you and assist you when difficult times arise.

Giving birth to a child is a very unique and personal experience, but it also has a universal and social tone as well. Family, especially the father, is and for the most part wants, to be part of the process. The grandmother also has a special role to play, having gone through this before, giving birth to you. Her wisdom can be invaluable, provided she can be guided to play her part without invading your privacy in ways you are not comfortable with. Finally, your closest friends can be given roles to play during your pregnancy and even more at the time of labor.

Psychic images from your dreams can often help you determine what role certain people are meant to play in the process of your pregnancy and labor. You could have a dream depicting a friend as an additional coach during your labor. This might not be something you had even conceived of, but upon further consideration, you might find that it is exactly what you need to feel taken care of.

One woman I know changed doctors during the seventh month of her pregnancy after a dream she had in which she did not feel her physician listened to her. She woke up feeling anxious, with the distinct wish to change her doctor. Her real appointment with the doctor was the following week. The actual visit turned out just like her dream and left her feeling distraught and generally uncomfortable about having this particular person deliver her baby. She decided to follow the hint from her dream even though her reason was telling her it was a stupid thing to do. After all, who had ever heard of changing doctors at the last minute? Making some inquiries, she found out that another woman she knew had had the same experience with the same physician and switched to a brand-new doctor very late in her pregnancy. She never regretted her decision. This convinced Celia that following the direction of her psychic dream was what she must do for her own peace of mind. In this way, the psychic dream gave her the additional boost she needed to follow her intuition. Without the dream she might not have dared to proceed with this drastic measure on the strength of her feelings about the visit alone. The new doctor turned out to be a perfect match for Celia. He was confident without being aggressive and nurturing without being controlling. They quickly established a good rapport effortlessly, and he did not let her down during a rather long and somewhat difficult labor.

Just as with any other dream, the most important element to pay attention to with a psychic dream is the feeling you are left with by the time the dream is over. The feelings you experience during and after the dream, as much as the story of the dream itself, give you the clues you can choose to act upon if need be.

It is hard to determine if you are having a psychic dream until it is reenacted in your waking life. The impact of the dream on your thought process, the clarity of its images, and your own intuitive feeling can all help determine if it is likely to be a premonition. If you feel moved to take the dream seriously and act upon it, then the implication is that the dream has a legitimate reason to exist. These dreams are different from anxiety dreams in that they are not directly threatening in the way an anxiety dream can be. They do not shake you up in the same way. They tend to be an affirmation of what is going right, or confirm feelings that you are already aware of on some level but have chosen to ignore until now. Many psychic dreams illuminate the consequences of actions you have thought about taking. Like a movie preview, they highlight what can happen according to your present state of mind. This does not mean that things are bound to happen the way they are shown in the dream. The psychic dream is a dream of possibilities or even probabilities. You are always the final arbiter of your own life. When you choose to change your mind-set, your future changes accordingly.

A psychic dream is an ally, a momentary insight into future probabilities. Use the information or dismiss it from your mind. In either case, do what feels right and trust your instinctual response to the dream images. The more you value these premonition dreams, the more they can become a natural part of your life and inform your most delicate decisions.

EXERCISE

The Power of Psychic Images

As you may have noticed, the psychic images in the dreams discussed in this chapter have their own role to play in the life of a pregnant woman. Even a dream that is purely psychic can have personal implications that are worth delving into in the context of pregnancy and labor.

This next exercise is geared toward exploring the ramifications and personal use of psychic dreams, such as finding a new anchoring image during labor, as well as checking in with your unconscious feelings about the approaching labor and the birth of your new baby.

Reviewing the Psychic Dream

• When a dream has come true in your daily life, go back and look at the dream again. If you are in the habit of writing your dreams down, this should not be a difficult process. If you have not done so, try to recall the dream by closing your eyes and letting your mind take you back into the atmosphere of the dream first without trying to get the right sequence of images. Very often what you remember first can be very informative and point to what struck you in the first place.

• Check for differences between the dream and the real-life event. What is the tone of the dream? Is the story exactly the same? How does it differ? What impact, if any, do the differences have on you emotionally?

Choosing a Psychic Image from the Dream

• Find the elements or symbols that stand out in your memory. Choose the images that move you the most and see if any of them can be of assistance to you for the rest of the pregnancy or for the labor. For instance, if you had a dream in which a dog was featured, like our first dreamer did, this image can turn out to be a valuable symbol for you. It is an image rich in meaning, a symbol of loyalty, friendship, protection, and the like. It might be the ideal anchor for you to use during the labor.

• Let the image inform you. Do not judge it or dismiss it too quickly. The intricate beauty of a spider's web can be just as nourishing an image as the joyous nature of a seal. In the web is reflected all the perfection of life's creation. This simple image is a graceful metaphor for the life being created inside the body of a woman, as another dreamer came to believe.

Checking In

Some psychic dreams also carry within them revelatory feelings, however unconscious they might be, regarding the labor and birth of the new child. These feelings get acted out in dreams and projected out into real life because they are not always pleasant or easy for the pregnant woman to accept in herself.

One woman had a dream in which her mother and her sister were having a fight in her kitchen. When she witnessed the same fight in her waking life just a few days later, it jolted her. She remembered her dream and saw that she had her own unresolved issues with her mother. Until now her younger sister had taken on the role of the rebellious one, but in the dream, she had experienced as much rage as her little sister, even though she was not the one fighting with her mother directly. The psychic dream gave her retrospectively the courage to face some of these feelings she had let her younger sister carry for her all these years.

If you believe that your dream might carry such revelations of unsavory emotions like rage, jealousy, or fear, do the following:

- Remember that you are not the only one going through this. Hundreds if not millions of other pregnant women have probably experienced some version or another of this particular feeling.
- Let go of judgment. Be thankful for the opportunity to look at the kind of energy you are carrying in your body.
- You have a choice: to honor it, accept it, let it go, channel it, change it, or all of the above.
- Give yourself a break. You do not have to take everything, even a psychic dream, so seriously. Dreams are clues, helpful allies, not sentences or jailers. Let them lead you to experience more freedom in your waking life.

CHAPTER SEVEN

Mystical Experiences

This chapter is in the book even though it does not include typical nighttime dreams because the women I interviewed believed as I do, that these visionary experiences were an extension of the premonitory quality of their dreams during their pregnancy. Moreover the transcendent quality of these occurrences had never been a part of these women's way of perceiving life until they either were pregnant or seriously considering becoming pregnant.

In this chapter we leave the conventional realm of interpretation and embrace a more spiritual connection with the world of souls who have not yet achieved a physical form but are already communicating their thoughts and wishes to the living.

The clarity and certainty of the women who had these experiences make their testimony stand on its own merit and are certainly worth recording. There is above all the sense that these women are uniquely connected to the spirit of their unborn child in a very particular way. Each woman allowed herself, in essence, to be guided or directed by this soul speaking to them from its invisible realm, and participated actively in the decision-making process of what house to move to, what clothes to buy, and so on. The women trusted this voice implicitly, recognizing it without the shadow of a doubt as the soul voice of their unborn baby.

A woman can go to great lengths in her determination to make a safe nest for her newborn. Many of the women interviewed chose to move into a new house during their second and third trimester at a time when it was very inconvenient to do so. What they also admitted was that they felt guided, even compelled, by the spirit of their unborn child not only to pack up and find a new home but also in the choice of the house itself.

In Stacy's case, the decision to move to a new house came after she and her husband had decided to "try to get pregnant." She had just gotten off the Pill, and expected that it would take her a while as it had for her friends. They had found what seemed to be the perfect house and decided to go into escrow. But Stacy felt uncomfortable, though she could not say why. They went back to look at the house again, and as they walked in, she remembers feeling a cold breeze on her neck and a sense of complete disapproval, as if someone was saying, "I hate this place. I'm not living here."

Meanwhile, the agent had told them about another house but that it was a waste of time to see it because other people already had a bid on it and it was almost a sealed deal. Stacy insisted that they must go and see it right away. As she would not take no for an answer (women who are in "nesting" mode can be very stubborn), they went along with her desire to see this unavailable house. The moment they walked in, Stacy felt at home. This was it. An acute feeling of joy coming from everywhere hit her heart with unmistakable precision, as if someone was saying to her, "This is my house! This is where I want to live." She walked into the backyard and was overcome with emotion. Like a vision, she saw herself with her child sitting under the shade of the tree, playing by the waterfall, chasing her hens and her old white cat, or using the swing installed between two trees at the other end of the yard by the bougainvilleas, next to the greenhouse a sculptor had obviously made his own, turning it into an artist's studio. All this she saw so clearly and the joy she felt wrapping itself around her was so palpable that she became convinced the spirit of her not-yet-conceived child was trying to make her realize that this was the home she wanted to be born into and that she would be happy here.

Stacy told the agent that this was their new home, that her baby wanted to be born here. Of course the agent thought she was not quite in her right mind, especially since the house was as good as sold. Stacy believed greater forces were at work and insisted that the agent call the owners again. The following day, the agent called, and with a certain degree of disbelief in her voice announced that the deal had fallen through and the house was theirs if they came up with an extra $10,000 beyond their original offer. Well, they did not have an extra penny to spare. They had put together everything they had to come up with a down payment but Stacy immediately said yes. When her husband looked at her like she had really gone mad, she just said that she would get it.

Three weeks later, the day the escrow was supposed to close, Stacy got a check in the mail for exactly $10,000. It was a residual check for a job she had done a year before. Two days after they moved into their new house, 3½ weeks after Stacy had stopped taking her birth control pills, their daughter was conceived. To this day, Stacy is firmly convinced that her daughter was behind everything, deciding where and when she wanted to come into this world and how to make that happen. "It was as if I could hear her talking to me inside my head and feel her presence all around me, touching my skin with her joy, or her reproach when I hesitated to listen."

No one except the woman experiencing it can fully understand what it is like to feel the almost palpable presence of your child around you long before you even carry it inside your own body. And yet scores of women have felt that exact presence with such startling conviction that no one could talk them out of it. They could just tell it was the spirit of their child making its presence known around them.

Susan's case is no exception. She was sitting in church at a Sunday service when she became aware of what she calls "a consciousness of pure love" floating all around her. Her immediate thought was: *This is my baby!* She sat there with tears streaming down her face. She had never considered having a child before—as a matter of fact, the idea terrified her—but the magnitude of the love pouring itself over her melted her fears away. It was too beautiful to ignore or not want to be part of. She accepted this love in her heart even though it was almost overwhelming for her, and became pregnant a year later.

During the second half of her pregnancy, Susan was shopping with a friend, not thinking about her baby. She remembers being in a very quiet mood, not talking, just musing around the store, which contained all kinds of things from soap to candles and even jewelry. It was one of those places you can come out of with a postcard or pretty writing paper you never intended to get in the first place. Susan wandered to the back of the store where they had a clothing section of pure cotton knits. She naturally picked up a pair of these "darling" cotton baby jumpers, and again was overcome by that exact same "consciousness of pure love" she had felt months earlier. And again the same thought came into her mind: *This is my baby*. It was such an extraordinary feeling that tears started streaming down her face as previously. She could not say anything to her friend; the experience was beyond words. So she stood there holding the baby jumper with wet cheeks, caught in the unfathomable love of her child, until she could move again.

Such mystical experiences are not uncommon among pregnant women. They connect women to their feminine nature in a very particular way. These visions give them an unusual frame of reference that is purely intuitive and yet completely real to the women who go through this type of experience.

Just like the dreams of the second and third

trimester, these visions can be put to good use for the labor and even help a woman adjust to the new relationship of mother and newborn. Sometimes they can have a beneficial influence on otherwise painful or difficult situations in real life.

In the transitional state between waking and sleeping, one woman had a vision that completely transformed her labor at its most crucial moment. At the time she could not tell whether she was dreaming or not, although there was a definite sense of "heightened perception" that filled her body with an odd passive alertness.

> *I am sitting in the center of a circle of women. One of them is the leader. She looks like a high priestess, dressed in a long hyacinth-blue robe and an odd-shaped hat, a sort of cone, the color of gold. She speaks to me in a silent language that I seem to understand perfectly. She takes the cone hat off and places it on my head. It is part of a ceremony. As soon as the hat is on my head, I begin to feel a great deal of warmth, and there is an incredible brightness enveloping me. I feel totally relaxed and filled with strength and power. It is an awesome feeling. The high priestess tells me this is her gift to me, part of my heritage as a woman, and that I must make good and timely use of it. I am not sure what she means by that. Everything fades from my perception, except that the feeling of this strange hat stays with me all day. It reminds me of an old sorcerer or magician's hat. It is an indescribable feeling of comfort and knowing that I am taken care of.*

Now comes the most amazing part of the story. During her very long and painful labor, which she was having with a midwife and no drugs of any kind, not even an epidural, this woman came to a place where she felt she could not handle the pain of the birth, which was transverse. She thought that at any moment the pain would run her over like a wild ox and kill her. It was the most unbearable, unnamable pain she had ever suffered. Her conscious mind could not fathom that a human being could endure such pain and not die. At that moment, she heard a voice that pierced through the veil of her agony so clearly she could not help but listen. It simply said to her, "Put the hat on." She knew instantly what the voice meant. Because she had nothing to lose, she started to visualize putting the golden cone on her head. She immediately experienced relief. Bathed in the golden light the hat radiated, she regained her composure. The pain dissipated completely. It remained but a shadowy memory of what it had been until she gave birth to her baby boy an hour later. In making this connection with her unconscious, she was able to tap into a source of power and comfort that was great enough to match her inhuman pain.

In fact, this vision was the only way she had to deal with the labor, and though she did not know it at the time, her psyche had provided her with the exact tools she needed in order to get through it. In this instance, it was a golden pointed hat, reminiscent of the head-dress Tibetan monks wear as well as other such ancient mystical beings as wizards and alchemists. Such is the power of dreams and visions, that they can provide almost instant relief or support in the most dire straits.

And such is the intuitive connection to life of pregnant women, that they can tap into a power hitherto unknown to them. The creative energy forming itself into their future child is identical to the life force running through their own being. This energy is the same energy that inhabits all things at the beginning of life, a concentration of such proportion as to bring about the birth of a whole universe. The making of a new human being is the result of a similar expansion of energy, the kind that creates a universe full of stars and galaxies, with its own laws and its own directive. Who is to say that such an event, filled with such immeasurable energy, could not also bring along with it the most beautiful and timely visions as well as the most accurate dreams of future events.

Mystical and psychic moments in our lives are reminders that we lead a spiritual life as well as a physical one. They create a path through which we can experience ourselves more fully. We are creatures whose imagination is as rich as the Milky Way. As a pregnant woman you can merge with the spiritual and earthly nature of things at the same time, for they are inextricably intertwined in the mystery of creation.

Do not dismiss the gifts or ignore the visions because they seem tenuous or fleeting. Do not be like Orual in C. S. Lewis's "Till We Have Faces," who disbelieves her brief vision of God's dwelling and, through her dismissal of it, betrays her sister Psyche's love. And on the other hand, do not feel that these visions are indispensable to your pregnancy. It is like going to a garage sale. Sometimes it is all crap and sometimes you discover a treasure. You keep going back because it is fun, and there is always the possibility of finding something unique and wonderful.

Each pregnancy has its own particular story, with its own journey. Just make sure that you live your pregnancy as fully and consciously as you can. Pregnancy is a time of transition, a preparation for motherhood. Your dreaming life is a tool and a gift that can enrich your experience and assist you in the transformation from girl/woman to mother/woman.

EXERCISE

Opening to the Visionary Aspect of Life

This exercise is geared toward opening yourself to the possibility of having visions in your life. The best way to approach this is to look at it as daydreaming, and then guiding the wanderings of your imagination through a specific intention or setting of a goal. As a young child you probably did this without thinking about it. You would be bored in class and look out the window and pretty soon you would be out there living a wild adventure in the woods, far, far from the classroom, until the teacher called on you or something else brought your attention back to the present reality.

In this exercise, you are essentially going to do the same thing as the child did, except you are going to set a specific intention or goal that will be the guiding force behind your daydreaming. It will give your wanderings a specific theme to focus on. In a way you will be your own oracle: The daydreams will answer the specific questions you have assigned them.

For instance, let us say that you would like to have a vision of what your child will be like seven years from now.

- Having a vision of your child when she/he is seven is the *specific intention* you are using to *focus* your imagination.
- Next, *let your eyes go out of focus* or look at a relatively distant landscape. You can look out the window or down at the floor. It needs to be something that does not require much effort. In other words, *you are looking without looking*.
- Begin to *daydream* about what your child would look like seven years from now.
- This part is optional but I highly recommend it. *Speak as if you were an Oracle*. Whatever comes to you in the daydream, however insignificant, *speak it out loud*:

"I see my son playing with his friends in the courtyard. He wears a red T-shirt and green shorts. It is his favorite get-up and it is quite worn and dirty. He is engrossed in a game of tag. His hair is wild and tousled and very dark. He runs faster than the other kids. He has this air of self-confidence about him, an effortless charm that strikes me. He is fierce, fair, and not afraid of his emotions."

As you can see, I have made this part quite detailed. Even if only one or two things come to you, make them as precise as you can. Have fun with it. Make it a positive experience for yourself. You will not regret it.

You can use this exercise for all sorts of things, not just for your child, but for yourself as well. Start small. Make sure you are comfortable with what you are daydreaming about. Do not fret about whether your daydream will become a reality. Let it go as soon as you have done it. This is just an exercise to open you up to the visionary aspect of your life.

We are all visionaries in one way or another. But not everything we daydream about comes true in our lives, which is a good thing. Personally, I do not have perfect dominion over my thought process, so I am very glad that some of my less-than-positive thinking does not come true!

Even with all its trials and tribulations, such as morning sickness, anxiety dreams about the health of the child, or about being a good enough mother or a different one from the kind of mother your mother was to you, even with the pain of the labor and the overwhelming feelings of responsibility, becoming a mother is a mystical experience.

The dreams and other visionary moments that occur during the nine months of pregnancy are part of the banquet served for you and only you at this particular time in your life. They are a window into the infinite love that can create the incomprehensible beauty of a newborn child.

And by the way, whether this can be termed "an old wive's tale" or not, for most of the women interviewed, the general consensus was that the more difficult and worrisome the dreaming life of the mother-to-be, the easier the labor and delivery of the baby turned out to be. So just think of your dreams as intense psychological and emotional preparation, with multiple possible scenarios so that when the actual labor occurs it is relatively easy and uneventful compared to your overactive dreamtime stories.

PART III

❦

Dreams
of the Father

❦

From dreams of the past to mystical experiences, the dreams of fathers-to-be are as vivid and poignant as those of their spouses. However, for this book, the dreams of the fathers-to-be come, for the most part, secondhand, through their wives. Whether out of shyness or diffidence, there was a certain resistance to the confessional nature of the interviews. This revealing of the most secret part of their psyche seemed to be distasteful to a great deal of the men involved. They were interestingly still willing to contribute and share their dreams but not in person. "You tell her. I already told you," was what the women were told. It is therefore mostly through the women that the dreams of fathers-to-be were reported to me. Very few spoke directly with me, so you and I have to trust their wives for an accurate retelling of their husbands' dreams.

It is interesting to note that the men followed a pattern that was consistent with the dreams of the women in the three phases of their pregnancy. For instance, in the first trimester, many of the fathers-to-be experienced dreams of the past, reacquainting themselves with their own childhood and dreams of lost love. There was often a feeling of guilt that accompanied the dreams about an ex-lover. They also had dreams of feeling trapped that were reminiscent of their initial fears about getting married.

During the second trimester of the pregnancy, the elation about being able to hear the child's heartbeat or feel his or her little kicks through touch translated into heroic dreams about saving everyone from the family dog to the whole world. Of course, anxiety dreams about protecting the child and about being a good enough father were also quite prevalent.

In the third trimester, dreams of labor and games of endurance seem to prevail. Several of the men experienced couvade symptoms in their dreams, as if they were going through the labor themselves. Of course, there were plenty of dreams about missing the birth of their child, especially among men with demanding schedules, and dreams in which, to his utter dismay, the man was put in the position of having to deliver his own baby.

The feeling that the men were part of a great mystery and did not have the right key to unravel or explain it often translated into dreams of being lost in some sort of cave or labyrinth in the dark. The general feeling was that they had entered somewhere they did not belong, like Indiana Jones or some other adventurer, and were only temporarily allowed in by virtue of their wives' condition.

Mystical and psychic experiences occurred in the fathers-to-be's dreams around the second trimester, which is congruent with the women's experience as well. Overall, the men seemed to be on the same dreaming schedule as their wives.

Of course, some of the future fathers did not just dream about their wives' pregnancy or labor; some of them actually experienced similar physical symptoms, like weight gain and even a little morning sickness, in a literal couvade fashion. This is a pretty rare experience, though.

CHAPTER EIGHT

Dreams of the Past

Finding out that you are going to be a father is an incredible revelation for a man. The experience is translated into dreams that run the gamut from great heroic acts to guilt-ridden sexual fantasies, from winning the lottery to being stuck at the epicenter of a massive earthquake.

Not only will the future father have to face himself, his fears about being a good enough father, or better than his own father, but he will also have to deal with the sense that everything is inevitably and forever changed. The new responsibility, the worry about being a good "provider," the desire to protect or to run away are all deep currents that pervade the dreamlife of the father-to-be. These currents appear all the more poignantly in the dreamscape of the future father because they often remain unexpressed in the waking life of the man. Deaming provides a safe avenue for the man to give difficult feelings a voice.

Father and Son

In many childhood dreams, the future father identified with the baby, remembering himself as the helpless babe and yet being the one caring for the baby at the same time. In this way the man is confronted with his own vulnerability as well as his capacity to nurture. This can be traumatic, especially if the man was raised by a very "male" father or someone who had difficulty showing his feelings. There can be a sense of loss of control, which, if correctly interpreted, is really an opening to new dimensions of character and literally an opening to new life.

This rediscovery of his own infant self was at the essence of a series of dreams Jason had. Thanks to the dreams, he was able to realize that it was up to him to take care of the future baby and that the baby needed him. He had been raised by a violent father and an absentee mother. During the first few months of his wife's pregnancy, through his dreams he reexperienced many of the feelings of fear and lack of safety he had as a child. Feelings of depression and shame surfaced, which he was able to acknowledge and talk about. He also went through a death and rebirth, letting go of the past and learning his own delight in nurturing an infant as this next dream shows:

> I am climbing down a hillside in Asia with an old and dear friend. There are small thatch-roofed

houses all around us, with small private yards. I watch my friend lie down in one of the yards and die. His body slowly dissolves into a swirl of black energy. After seeing him do this, I also decide to lie down. Instantly my body begins to come apart into a thousand pieces of pulsing darkness and slowly I too fade into death. When I awake I am lying in a large bed with silk sheets. A beautiful baby boy is handed to me. I hear a voice that tells me the child is my son. He looks just like me. The baby feels safe in my arms because he knows that I have died and come back to life. My level of experience enables the baby to trust me. He holds on to me even tighter than before, afraid to let go and be on his own. I feel good holding my son. I wake up.

There are many interesting elements in this dream of the past that work together to create a perfect tool for the dreamer. First, his old friend shows him the way, so to speak, by dying first. He is being shown the end of his old life. He follows suit and finds himself waking up in a silk bed and being handed this baby. A voice tells him that this is his son. So something as final as death turns out to be the bringer of new life. Notice that the friend is not part of the second half of the dream; he remains dead. There has been a drastic change in the life Jason used to live. Because his son knows that *he has died and come back to life*, he feels safe with his father. There is a definite element of myth in this dream. The theme of the hero having to go into the underworld and come back from the dead is prevalent in many stories with both male and female heroes.

Not only did Jason feel that he had to "die to his old life" in order to become a father, but he also felt that he had to "die to his own childhood" and let go of the past, the way it was for him, in order to embrace a new way. Another equally interesting factor in the dream is that the child is a son who looks just like him. Without adhering to the notion that all characters in dreams are aspects of ourselves, it is clear that the son in the dream is the part of Jason that he is now able to love and to nurture, no matter what. This is emphasized in another dream that occurs later on. In it, Jason is carrying his son who turns into a wolf-type beast, and yet he is still willing to cherish and keep the child who is holding onto him for dear life. This dream shows a level of acceptance and a capacity to nurture even the shadow side of his own nature. This openness had not been present or at least not available to Jason until now.

Many dreams involving father and son seem to pervade the dreamscape of fathers-to-be during the early part of their wives' pregnancies. These dreams often include symbols that offer a recapitulation of their own relationship with their father, as well as an opportunity to embrace the child part of themselves in a more tender and open way. Becoming a father is a time when a man can get in touch with his capacity to nurture.

Ex-Lovers and Fantasies

Though men dream about ex-lovers just as frequently as women in their first trimester, their dreams are generally not as violent or rich in death symbolism as the women's dreams seem to be. I am sure hormones have something to do with it. However, I believe that the men's dreams about ex-lovers tend to converge toward a more sexual direction. Missed opportunities and erotic fantasies are layered over previous encounters with other women, creating a rich, sexually oriented landscape that is uniquely male and encapsulates the feeling that their erotic days are over. Of course, many women are very sexual during their entire pregnancy, so these dreams are more often based on fear than truth, but they feed the illusion that becoming a father means a desexualization of the relationship. Frankly, for me personally, I think it would be a matter of practicality, whether the size of my body and my control over the distribution of the weight would allow me enough freedom of movement to enjoy sex!

In this next dream, the father-to-be ends up rejecting a sexual fantasy, a ménage à trois, in order to take care of a baby, which he finds surprisingly fulfilling and rewarding in a way that brings him a lot of joy.

> *I am in my older brother's bedroom watching television. Two women who are my brother's ex-girlfriends want to take care of me. I am feeling turned on and guilty at the same time. A baby is crying in the next room. I get up and walk into the next room. A bald and smiling baby with shiny eyes greets me with his arms reaching up to me. I pick him up. I change his clothes. I feel incredibly happy to be taking care of him. I feel good all over. I wake up.*

The setup at the beginning of the dream is reminiscent of adolescence: a young man hanging out with his older brother, watching television. The sexual competition with his brother is portrayed in the dream by the two women being ex-girlfriends of the older brother. When the baby is heard crying in the next room, however, the father-to-be feels compelled to leave his fantasy behind.

This fantasy is also a fantasy of the past, which in reality was not really as much fun as the dream. There was a lot of competitiveness between the brothers, and our future father often felt inferior, not as accomplished as his handsome, athletic older brother. Given the opportunity to fulfill his fantasy in his brother's bed, Mark finds himself choosing to respond to the call of the baby in the next room and abandon his fantasy, which, upon reflection, did not feel all that wonderful.

There was a sense of guilt in this first part of the dream that interfered with his enjoyment of the situation. He realized he still had some unresolved feelings left over from an affair he did have with an ex-lover of his brother. It had created a gulf between them that had taken a long time to mend.

The dream gave a chance to Mark to come to terms with the past and realize that what he was moving toward was just as satisfying as an erotic fantasy, but in a different way.

Dreams of the past allow the psyche to adjust to the new future at hand. Dreams of childhood, reconnecting with the roles of both child and father, prepare the man to become a father. They can also give voice to anxieties about repeating the mistakes of the father and help the father-to-be through deep feeling waters that are brought to the surface by his wife's pregnancy.

Some Helpful Hints

• Sharing these types of dreams with your wife will help you realize that she is actually going through similar feelings and worries that come out in her dreaming life as much as they do in yours.

• If you begin early on to establish a dialogue about your respective dreams, it will help your level of intimacy throughout the pregnancy and give you a greater feeling of participation for the whole duration.

• Dreams are the language of the soul. They assist you in this crucial transition into fatherhood. They show you a way to heal old wounds so that you can grow to become the father you want to be. They are full of self-discoveries.

• Do not be selfish. Help each other understand your respective night stories. Sometimes a person who knows you well can understand the metaphors of your dreams more easily than you can because you are too close to it.

• Another wonderful and helpful thing to do is to start a fathers-to-be group. If you do not know any fathers-to-be, ask your wife. She is probably involved in a pregnant women's group of some kind, prenatal yoga class, or the like and these women may have partners you could get in touch with.

• Talk about your dreams, day ones as well as night ones. Discuss your elation and your fears. If you get support, it will be easier for you to be there for your wife when she really needs you.

• Find out special things you can do to help your wife during the last trimester and the labor. Get a midwife to come and give a talk to your group. Start the group as early on in the pregnancy as you can and keep tabs on each other.

• Celebrate each man's transition into fatherhood. Exchange stories; do not just pass out the cigars. Find out from a new father what it was like to go through the labor with his wife. Get a man who you consider to be a "good father" to come and share his experience of fatherhood with your group.

• Have fun. Living with an increasingly pregnant wife and the imminent arrival of your child has its humorous moments.

EXERCISE

Father and Son

If you have dreams that bring up anxiety about becoming a father or relate to your own childhood, do the following exercise:

• Take a specific situation from your childhood.
• Remember yourself as clearly and in as much detail as possible.
• Make a list that includes the following:
  Age: I am eight years old and proud of it.
  Appearance: I am skinny. I have a bruised knee. I am wearing a torn sweatshirt and black trousers and sneakers.
  Attitude: I am looking down at a pebble, defiantly ignoring my father's command to look at him when he talks to me.

Feelings: I am scared.

- Remember your father in as much detail as you did yourself.
- Run the situation/incident through your mind. It should not be too hard. Some events stick to our brains so vividly we can never forget them even if we want to. Hopefully this is one of those. Make sure you have the sequence down before you start playing around with it.
- Now put yourself in your father's shoes. Become the father to the eight-year-old you once were.
  What would you do differently?
  What would you do the same?
  How would you relate to the eight-year-old?

If you do this exercise thoroughly and honestly, you might come up with some very useful information about yourself and some poignant revelations about your relationship with your father.

After you have done this first half of the exercise, find a second situation that has left a wonderful memory, or at least a loving memory, of your relationship with your father. It should be the kind of memory you hope you will have with your own child someday. Follow the same steps as with the first exercise. This part of the exercise is a healing process and gives a sense of closure, or at least completion, to the whole sequence. It is a powerful tool if your relationship to your own father has left you with a lot of emotional residue, the kind of stuff that could get in the way of your own relationship with your child.

Trust the process; observe where it takes you. Take some notes. Sometimes it helps to write things down.

You might want to keep your own dream journal during the whole pregnancy and track the evolution of your dreams and the feelings that arise from them. Share what you believe is important with your wife. It will help you stay in touch with the fact that you are playing an integral part in the pregnancy. Without you, this would not be happening.

CHAPTER NINE

From Hero to Background Player

By the second trimester, many fathers-to-be have begun to realize that "this is for real . . . there really is a baby growing in there." For many, this is a time of jubilation. "I am going to be a father!" becomes the mantra that runs through their minds day and night; the ecstasy and the agony of it settles in their psyche, leaving fresh and indelible marks that give rise to fertile dream activity in the most reluctant dreamers.

For some of these fathers-to-be, heroic deeds become a fixture of their dreaming landscape. For others, their dreams center around the sexual organ, prominently featured and worthy of worship in its obvious fertility. The heroes these fathers-to-be identify with might have changed from John Wayne to Bruce Willis, Jackie Chan, or Denzel Washington, but the tone is the same. However, these heroic men, like the women, do not escape the anxiety dreams that can plague the second trimester and sometimes overtake the bravest father-to-be's dreaming life. The anxiety dreams can be accompanied by feelings of being expendable, as the mother-to-be cocoons herself around her experience of inner bonding with the baby. To be reminded of the love that created this child can be all the reassurance a father-to-be needs. It is easy enough for a wife to do this, but if she does not, then it is the father's responsibility to ask her for it.

Heroism and Celebration

Heroes come in all shapes and sizes. One man, as his wife reported, began having consistent heroic dreams where he would be Spiderman one night, Batman the next, always saving women, or the world in general, from destruction. These dreams left him both elated and exhausted. Battling evil every night, he had become the protector on an archetypal level. One of the most interesting characters he identified with in his most prominently recurring dream was the character Jean Reno played in the film *The Professional*. Well, in his dreams, Mark was The Professional, the good-bad guy who ends up protecting a twelve-year-old girl and dying for her. Mark really saw his role as husband and father-to-be as this protector archetype.

What his subconscious was really asking for was to be thanked for his efforts to be a good husband and his hard work to bring a bigger paycheck home for his expanding family. He also needed to be reminded that he did not have to be perfect and invincible, that he could be human and scared.

Some of the heroic deeds in Mark's dreams masked a great deal of anxiety about his ability to be a good enough father. This anxiety subsided as he accepted his human limitations, which were essential to balance out his superdad complex. He was trying to live up to an impossible and unreal image of what his unconscious mind believed his own father had been.

Another heroic father-to-be concentrated his dreaming art on an old childhood fantasy, being a firefighter. Nick had always wanted to be a firefighter when he was a child. When his wife became pregnant, he started living out this old fantasy in his dreams on a regular basis. Putting out fires, saving children and dogs from raging flames, became his nightly occupation. For Nick these dreams were very empowering and thrilling. He felt as if he had gotten in touch with a new strength he had not known he possessed before.

Fire itself is a fascinating element. There are stories of firefighters setting their own fires in order to be able to save people. Pyromaniacs worship fire in their own dangerous way. "Don't play with matches" is probably one of the first serious admonitions told to a child.

As a symbol, fire is not only destructive but purifying. It leaves the landscape forever changed, but also promotes new growth, new life rising from the ashes. Fire is a powerful enemy, but when tamed, it represents the center of the hearth, cooks our food, and keeps us warm. Storytelling always occurs around the campfire. And since the beginning of time it was regarded with respect as an instrument of God's power.

This brings me to the two major themes that are

consistently present in all the heroic dreams of a father-to-be and that could not exist without each other. On the one hand, there is the heroic aspect of the dream, which is what the father-to-be becomes identified with, a hero, and on the other hand, there is what he battles with, usually natural elements, such as fire, earthquakes, or floods, from which he rescues women, children, and pets. The energy that infuses him with heroic capabilities is the same energy that he is battling in these fires and other disasters. It is the energy of creation, of new life.

The knowledge that he is going to become a father, as well as witnessing the transformation of his wife, galvanizes his very being with renewed passion for life. In his dreams, he becomes the hero. In a way he is compelled to become this larger-than-life figure because he is dealing with something that is larger than his own life, larger than anything he has ever experienced before, the creation of his child. This creative power is the same power he becomes embattled with in his dreams. This creative energy is the energy of fire and flood; it is the energy of life itself in all its awfulness and grandeur. The mystery is unfolding and the man is caught in it, even if he does not fully understand it or even accept it.

Recognition of this ineluctable process of nature makes its appearance in dreams where the father-to-be exhibits his private parts in a contest of some kind of which he is the unmistakable winner. The penis has been worshiped in one form or another for thousands of years. In these celebratory dreams, the penis takes on its best and most appropriate role as a potent symbol of fertility and love rather than the search-and-destroy meaning of deadly nuclear bombs.

Birthday parties are another common theme for the dreams of fathers-to-be. They express the idea of change as well as celebration. It is no accident that the word *birth* is part of this theme since it implies that something is being given birth to here: not only the baby, but indeed the birth of a new father as well. They are being born together, just like mother and child are giving birth to each other. The rich symbology of dreams conveys this mutually transformative pattern very well through these triumphant and celebratory dreams.

The Anxiety of the Background Player

Another trend in the dreams of future fathers appears toward the end of the second trimester, often unexpectedly. In many ways these dreams mimic the mothers-to-be's anxiety dreams. Some of the themes run parallel, like the fear-based dreams about the health and nature of the baby. Other dreams have a specific character that is more directly related to men. These dreams have to do with feeling unimportant or not essential to the process. The future father turns from hero into background player in his own dreaming arena, without realizing that these dreams reflect real feelings of displacement, abandonment, and worry about the future of his marriage.

These types of dreams are a direct reaction to the assumption that because a woman is more involved with her bonding process with the child she is carrying or getting ready for the birth, she does not appreciate the contribution her husband is making or is purposely ignoring him.

There are several ways to remedy this situation. The woman can reassure her husband that she indeed appreciates his efforts to make her life easier, make more money, find a new home, and so on. She can also make time for the two of them to have some fun together, like take a walk, cuddle in bed, watch a comedy, read the funnies together and the like. The man can choose to make the pregnancy a priority in his own life and be more directly involved in buying the crib, getting the room ready, learning about the different phases of labor, what his wife is going through physically, hormonally, and so on.

To be actively involved in the pregnancy is a great way to deal with the various anxieties and fears that can plague the dreaming life of a father-to-be. It gives an outlet to emotions and feelings that can otherwise be overwhelming.

The next two dreams illustrate the intensity of the feelings that can be present in the night stories of fathers-to-be. From rescuing his children from floods to being kept out of his own home, the husband of the mother-to-be is deeply involved in the process of becoming a father. His own psyche is helping him deal with this psychological and emotional adjustment in a rather dramatic fashion.

First dream:

> I come home and I find that the children are missing. They have been kidnapped. My wife is missing too. I have never been so terrified in my

life. I wake up. I feel so relieved this was just a dream. But it felt so real at the same time. I get up and walk around and check on the kids and everything. My wife wakes up. We talk a bit. She tells me she has had similar dreams. For some reason this reassures me more than anything.

With a third child on the way, this father-to-be felt an enormous pressure to provide a good environment for his whole family. He felt overwhelmed by the pressure of being up to the task. The standards he had set for himself were worthy of Hercules, that is to say, of heroic proportions. The result, however, was that he found himself feeling depressed, overworked, and alone. In the dream this is exemplified by the fact that all the people he is working so hard to protect and provide for have disappeared. Everything has been taken away from him in one fell swoop. The intense anxiety and terror he experiences wakes him up. After he had had a chance to take the dream in, he realized that he was so obsessed with "doing the right thing" that he was missing out on his life with his family. He was missing out on his children, his wife, and the pregnancy. Once balance was reestablished between work and home, the anxiety dreams lessened. He also began to participate in the process of "getting ready for the new baby" in a way he had not been able to before.

Second dream:

I am at the front door of this house. I know it is my house but it looks different at the same time.

I know my wife is getting ready to give birth in there. I want to come in and help her. I am bringing home these birthday presents. I have been working hard to get them. For some reason my key does not open the door. I feel angry that I cannot get into my own house. I start banging on the door, then screaming. But nothing happens, so I walk all around. I think I am going to have to climb up the fire ladder, up to the second floor window. I feel stupid, embarrassed, like a thief or a burglar. What if a neighbor saw me and thought I was a burglar? I am determined to get in even if I have to sneak in. I wake up.

This is another dream that is pretty self-explanatory. The father-to-be is bringing home presents for a birthday. It is not clear in the dream whose birthday it is, but there is a definite sense of coming home to celebrate a birth. When the father-to-be wants to get into the house, he is not able to do so. It is as if access has been denied or forbidden to him. He feels frustrated, angry, humiliated. The feelings are reminiscent of being left out of the game in the schoolyard. He is not with the "in" crowd. Another interesting thing to pay attention to is the fact that the house looks like his house and at the same time it is not his house. The home has become a symbol for the feminine mystery from which the man feels completely excluded. In fact, he is afraid of being taken for a burglar or a thief. It is almost as if a part of this future father knows that he cannot participate in certain rituals because they are foreign to his masculine nature. He feels excluded from the central mystery of childbirth; the only way he can see it is by sneaking like a thief into his house.

To feel shut out of the pregnancy is a common theme in the dreams of future fathers, whether it is true in their waking lives or not. It is an ancient emotion for men, and although the practices have changed and men participate much more actively in the pregnancy and birth process, there is still the prevalent notion, which comes through in their dreams, that future fathers are being allowed into a mysterious territory that is the domain of the feminine principle of life. Their dreams are filled with images showing the men as intruders or background players who protest their fate, knowing that something awesome is going on just beyond their reach.

Between the hero and the background player, there is a place the future father can come to rest, where he does not need to shoulder all the glory or all the responsibilities for the birth of his child, where he does not need to feel rejected, ignored, abused, overworked, or overwhelmed.

The second trimester—after the exhilaration and panic of the first trimester have settled down—is the perfect time to get some perspective. This next exercise is a useful tool at this juncture for all fathers who experience recurring anxiety dreams.

EXERCISE

Centering and Pregnancy

Take some time for yourself. It is probably the most important thing you can do. To relax, breathe deeply and allow all the feelings you are holding onto very tightly to loosen up. Trying not to feel what you are feeling is the best way to hold onto those very feelings.

- Choose a particular dream to work with, one that has left you with feelings of anxiety or worry.
- Instead of trying to figure out what the dream means, take the feelings from the dream and see how they apply to your waking life.
- Scan various situations the dream could apply to: work, relationship, your wife's pregnancy.
- Be as honest as you can. This is an exercise just for you.
- Pick one area where the feelings are the most concentrated. Let us say that what concerns you most is feeling left out of the process your wife is going through with the pregnancy. Besides feeling left out, check what other feelings this brings up for you:
- Do you feel alone, angry, worried, concerned?
- Do these feelings remind you of any other previous situation? Is it a recurring theme in your life?

Once you have a grasp of the feelings that are running through you, take a deep breath, hold it for a count of ten, and then release it. It is important not to tighten yourself up around these feelings, however uncomfortable they are. On the contrary, try to feel yourself opening and expanding around them. When you give your feelings room and acknowledge their existence, you are giving yourself room at the same time, room to go outside your circle of anxiety and worry.

The next step is the most important one: Make the pregnancy the center of your attention. Shift the focus from anxiety and worry to what is being created right now at this precise point in time inside the body of your wife. Imagine yourself as a witness of the coming into being of your child at this very moment. Something is happening, regardless of your worry or anxiety, something much greater than any computer you can ever manufacture, something beautiful that would not have come into existence without you.

Focus all of your attention on this intricate life that is part you, part her, part other, and so new it is not quite complete yet. Let the worry fall away like an old coat, and wrap yourself in the glory of this beautiful new life you have helped create. Stay with this feeling until it saturates your mind with its calm radiance.

The male spirit feels most happy and free involved in an action that requires its full attention. In this way he can experience the feeling of "rest in motion," which is similar to meditation, yet different from it in that it does not require "being still and thinking nothing." A father-to-be can experience the same sense of "rest in motion" if he allows himself to fully engage emotionally, psychologically, and physically in the pregnancy and the birth process. His dreaming life is not trying to be a source of worry and anxiety, but rather it is showing the future father ways in which he can participate more completely during the whole nine months it takes to create his child. The dreams are exploring aspects of fatherhood still developing in the man. The part of him that feels like the hero, the protector, the one left out of the feminine mystery—all these aspects are being worked through in the dreaming landscape. By bringing a conscious awareness to these dreams without judging them or simply dismissing them as anxiety dreams, a father-to-be uses his own inner wisdom to become more whole, to balance his nurturing self with his conquering spirit. The tenderness of a father as he holds his newborn is both fierce and gentle. And the awkwardness of his great love for this child is as beautiful as a mother's bond to her baby.

CHAPTER TEN

Dreams of Labor and Birth

In the last trimester before the birth of his child, a father-to-be experiences many dreams that relate directly to the labor and birth. In this way, again, there are similarities with the mother-to-be's own dreams in which she rehearses the labor. For the father-to-be dreams of labor often include couvade symptoms, in which he goes through some form of the labor himself. In certain dreams, the future father might be both the one giving birth as well as the doctor assisting the birth. In other dreams, the father might know that his wife is giving birth but not be able to participate in it. Or he may be prevented from getting there in time for the child's arrival. Some fathers also dream of being lost in caves or labyrinths, and others experience dreams in which they are put through tests that require immense endurance. These dreams are reminiscent of the heroic dreams of the second trimester. The main difference is that these dreams seem to concentrate specifically on endurance-type games of which they do not know the rules and the referee is part of a mystery they cannot solve.

One particular dream stands out that refers precisely to this "not knowing." In it, a father-to-be asks the teacher of the Lamaze class, "How are babies born?" This dream occurred the night before the future father and his pregnant wife were to attend their last natural childbirth session together. There is something poignant and funny about this very honest and child-like question, and yet it puts forth the mystery of birth in a very clear and succinct fashion. Here is this man who has dutifully showed up to learn how to help his wife go through the birth process and still he does not know any more than he did before he took his first lesson.

The dream of this father-to-be acknowledges how little we truly know, even with all of our technical prowess, about the mystery of birth. The innocence of the man's question is a recognition and an acceptance of this mystery, which actually shows an instinctual respect and unconscious understanding worth all the scientific answers in the world.

The overwhelming feelings of the father-to-be, as the date of the birth grows near, are very apparent in this following series of dreams. This future father had several dreams in a row right up until the time of the actual labor when he finally slept like the proverbial baby.

First dream:

> *I just know it is time, but I cannot find my keys.*
> *I am afraid my wife is going to have the baby*
> *right there at our doorstep. I start breathing very*
> *fast, a sort of hyperventilation/Lamaze thing. I*
> *wake up in a sweat.*

In this dream, the father-to-be is not in control of
the situation. He has "lost his keys. " His masculine
energy cannot work here. He is worried about the baby
coming at a time when he is not quite ready. The fact
that he is afraid that the baby will arrive at "his
doorstep" could be interpreted two ways. One is that
the baby is arriving at his doorstep. In other words, our
future father cannot deny the imminent arrival of his
child anymore. It is a fait accompli. The second interpretation refers to the imminence of the labor itself,
which was supposed to be happening any day in real
life. Finally, there is the added element of couvade in
his hyperventilation, which is reminiscent of the
Lamaze technique which he himself refers to. In other
words, the future father takes on the breathing technique of his wife during labor and wakes up in a sweat.

The next dream illuminates with even more intensity the father's concerns about the baby's arrival and
his lack of control. It also adds a humorous element.

Second dream:

> *I am in a dark tunnel of some kind. I have no*
> *idea where I am. My wife is in there with me.*
> *She seems to know what is going on, but I cer-*
> *tainly do not. I also do not see where she is. I*

feel uneasy, like something is wrong. I have to find her. I think she is in danger. There is a rival I have to meet. I am shocked because I have never felt this feeling of having a rival before. I wake up thinking about the arrival of our baby, which is due any day now.

There is a wonderful use of pun in this dream. It has to do with the words *a rival*. One of the elements these words stand for is the sense that a new being is entering the life of the couple, someone whom the husband finds threatening. He says, "I am shocked because I have never felt this feeling of having a rival before." He is definitely disturbed by this. What this aspect of the dream also symbolizes is in the words themselves: *a rival*, which is also *arrival*. The sound and spelling of these two words are so similar that it is unmistakably an association the unconscious mind of the husband has made on purpose. The *arrival* of the baby is also the *arrival* of *a rival*. And though the future father might not feel this way consciously, a part of him definitely experiences the baby's birth as a threat. The journey through the dark tunnel with no clear bearings, his wife knowing what is going on while he is lost and uneasy— all these elements of the dream combine to make a powerful picture of a future father who is ill at ease with the imminent changes in his relationship.

In this last dream before his wife went into labor, the father-to-be got a close look at the mystery of birth and his participation in it. It is probably a closer look than he wanted to get, a dream rich in symbolism, a final gift of preparation his own psyche wanted to give him before the actual birth of his child.

Third dream:

> *I am in a white room. At first I like how neat
> and clean everything is. I think I am alone but I
> am not sure. I start to feel as if I am being
> watched. I realize that I am in a hospital. The
> doctor, dressed in white, is with me, except he
> changes. He does not look like a real doctor
> anymore, more like a witch doctor. The room
> starts to change too. It's not white anymore. I
> worry about my wife. She must be in labor. I
> must go to her, help her with her breathing, hold
> her hand, encourage her, and all that. Instead,
> the next thing I know, I am on a table with this
> witch doctor doing his passes over me. It is really
> weird. He seems to be encouraging me. I just
> want to get the hell out. Next thing I know, I am
> standing in front of my wife; my hands are filled
> with blood. There are people screaming. Actu-
> ally it's me. I am screaming louder than even my
> wife is. There is a baby coming out. It is not nice
> at all. I feel sick to my stomach, embarrassed. I
> wake up thinking this is awful, not at all the pic-
> ture I had in my mind. Too gritty, gruesome,
> bloody. Not like on TV, that is for sure.*

There are several unusual motives in this last dream,
certainly a lot of reversals, such as the husband
becoming the patient, then taking the role of his wife
briefly, then becoming the doctor, then delivering the
baby, and so on. There is a gradual transformation of
the landscape from an antiseptic white room, with a
doctor in white, to a scene filled with screams, blood,

all orchestrated by a witch doctor, formerly the doctor in white. Something is taking over, something magical. The witch doctor makes passes over the father-to-be. He is suddenly the one on the bed. What is he encouraged to do? We can infer from the circumstances of the dream that this is actually the beginning of a couvade scene, with the husband taking on the role of his wife in labor. She is, after all, supposed to be next door going through the labor. This is confirmed in the next reversal when the husband has now become the doctor delivering his own baby. But instead of a dramatic but idyllic scene, what greets the dreamer is his own fear and horror at the griminess and bloodiness of the birth itself. It is as if the dreamer peered through the veil and got a glance at the nature of life. It was not what he expected. His clinical view of his personal involvement in the labor, i.e., hold his wife's hand, breathe with her, and so on, has been swept away by the unconscious landscape of his dream. In his dream, this father-to-be got to take a look at the feminine aspect of birth up close and personal. He got a chance to face his fears about it as well and to reassess his involvement.

The night his wife started her labor, he actually slept like a baby. And so did she. In fact, she decided to go back to sleep because she knew the birth would not be happening for a long time. She does not recall how much of the labor she slept through, but once they got to the hospital, it took less than three hours.

Her husband is convinced that she felt safe and relaxed because he had already gone through hell with the labor in his dreams! Maybe he is right.

During the third trimester men often get exhilarated

by the sense that they are in the home stretch, and yet they also feel caught in what appears to them to be a game of endurance or a waiting game. A part of them wants to know when this is going to be over. God forbid the date chosen by the doctor for the onset of labor passes without the slightest sign of a contraction.

Future fathers would be surprised to find out how many women feel exactly the same way. Generally, though, these feelings are more often expressed in dreams rather than shared verbally. This would be the perfect time to take advantage of that fathers-to-be group, which was hopefully started early in the first trimester.

Both men and women need support to go through this huge change in their lives. It is the most natural thing in the world and the most extraordinary. It is a matter of life and death, the death of the old life and the birth of a new life, a new family. Scary or funny, muddy or bright, our dreams are full of pearls to be gleaned for an expanded, more inclusive vision of our lives as lover, husband, wife, father, mother, and whatever other roles we choose to play in this lifetime.

EXERCISE

Labor Coach

Besides taking the Lamaze classes or other natural birth methods you have decided upon, the best way to prepare yourself for your wife's labor is to go through it, not literally of course, but to imagine yourself going through every step and to give yourself the capacity to be your wife's healer/witch doctor like the father did in the previous dream.

In this way, you are consciously contributing to your dreaming life. You are expanding it by using your imagination as a tool for transforming daydreams or wishful thinking into a potent activity of your mind. The tools you are using are simple. Essentially they are your desire to help and love.

Here Is How It Works

• Get informed about what to expect. Ask a father who hung in there with his wife every step of the way, someone who is honest, to tell you his experience. He might tell you that it was the most incredible experience of his life. He might also tell you that it was terrifying, that he could not bear to look. Many otherwise courageous men cannot deal with the blood and the screams of pain that women go through during the birthing process. He might say that the baby's arrival makes you forget everything else.

• Get the medical, objective point of view as well. It helps to know what "phase" you are entering into.

• Take the time to digest this information. Share it with fellow fathers-to-be.

• Once you feel that you have taken in as much information as you can and that you cannot get any more without going through the process itself, ask yourself what kind of role you would like to play in your wife's labor.

• What would you like your contribution to be?

• How do you see being able to make a difference?

• Do you want to be able to help her with her pain?

- Do you want to be able to protect both your wife and your baby during the whole process?

Setting the Stage

- Let us say you want your wife and baby to feel protected by you during the labor. Give yourself a space of time when you can be quiet and relax.
- Read something that makes you feel at peace and calms your mind. It can be anything, as long as it works for you, the Bible, *Sports Illustrated*, poetry by you. Listening to a piece of music or a song you love can produce the same effect. If taking a bath or running or roller blading does it for you, then do that. Do not watch television. It has the wrong sort of hypnotic effect and it does not relax you.

Your Body of Love

After you have completed your chosen activity, close your eyes for a moment to gather yourself and draw your attention inward.

Do not make this part of the exercise more difficult than it is. First off, use your imagination to create in your mind's eye as vivid a picture as you can of the labor. Think of this exercise as an alternative to one of your night stories about labor. Think of it as a waking dream, a conscious imaginary experience to express the power of your love during labor.

Ask yourself as many questions as you can to fill in the blanks: Where are you? At what stage is your wife in her labor? What is going on? Who is there? Doctor? Nurse? Are you next to your wife? What are your actions? What are you thinking and feeling? How is she doing? Is there a monitor with your baby's heartbeat that you can hear?

If your dreams about the labor are filled with helpless worry and if you want your wife to feel protected and held through this event, if you wish you could do more, then imagine the love that you feel as a real tangible thing. Feel the solidity of your body, the aliveness that is contained within it in every cell. Then take that feeling of pure aliveness and make it into a second body, like a ghost image coming out of you, shining with light, a body made of pure love, all the love you have ever experienced in your life, the love that was given to you and the love that you have given. Know that this body is also filled with all the power of your love for your wife and baby. Now let your body of light extend its arms and wrap around your wife.

Set the intention for your body of love to have a healing and protective effect on your wife and child. Make it so in your mind until it becomes so real you could take a picture of it.

Believe that this love can alleviate both your fear and her pain. Also hold your baby in this same love while he/she is making his/her transition from the world of the womb to the world of mother and father.

The love of a man and a father is strong and powerful, though different in quality than the love of a woman and a mother. It has a great deal of potential to heal, nurture, and protect. To love does not make you helpless. During labor it can be your most valuable asset. Let the body of your conscious dreaming help you hold your wife in the invisible arms of your love.

CHAPTER ELEVEN

Psychic Dreams and Other Mystical Experiences

Expecting a child is a life-changing experience for men as well as women, and the intuition of a future father blossoms during the time of his partner's pregnancy. There are uncanny similarities in the patterns of psychic dreams between men and women, as if they were on parallel courses. There are instances of psychic dreams in which the father-to-be, just like the future mother, meets their unborn child, experiences their personality, and recognizes their gender. The interpretation of the dream is not always accurate, but the dream itself is.

A man's intuition is not limited to the experience of their child's personality or sex. Some of the men who shared their night stories spoke of ancient rituals, like naming ceremonies. Others felt the presence of their child's spirit long before it was conceived. And some underwent a complete transformation of their lives spiritually, emotionally, and materially through the arrival of their child.

Some of these men truly moved through mystical events, as touching and profound as anything the women experienced. The impact and ramifications of their child's arrival was deeply felt through every fiber of their being. *Unexpected* and *exciting* were some of the words I heard about these premonitions and visionary dreams, both for the men who remembered them and the women who got a chance to witness the more intuitive sides of their husbands.

The Case of Mistaken Identity

The following dream is a fascinating example of a perfectly good psychic dream that reveals the sex and personality of the baby to the dreamer who then dismisses it or rather does not trust it because of cultural conditioning and social bias:

> *Toward the end of the second trimester, this father-to-be dreams of a baby with a sweet disposition. He sees this beautiful baby, laughing in its crib, looking up at him trustingly. With dark eyes fringed with long lashes and big black curls all over his head, the child tells the father that he is a boy.*

When the father woke up from the dream, he decided that the dream was wrong, that with such curly dark hair and long lashes the baby must be a girl. So he interpreted the curls as belonging to a girl. What is truly amazing is that the father-to-be did not deny the images from the dream—the dark curls, the eyes—but he denied the sex of the baby. For him curly hair, a sweet smile, and long eyelashes belonged to a girl.

When the baby was born, the father then realized how right on his dream had turned out to be and how prejudiced his interpretation of it had been, to the point where he had denied the truth spoken in the dream. This man had a psychic dream that was spot on, but his assumptions, formulated by social and familial conditioning, made him lean against the evidence provided by the dream. He chose to ignore the dream until he was faced with his newborn child. He realized that his baby boy with his beautiful dark curls was perfect, intent on being himself right from the start, and that he better start accepting this new little being right now. It was not only a simple psychic dream, but a powerful lesson as well.

The Naming Ceremony

In many traditions, from ancient Rome to Native American to Jewish mysticism, the naming of a child is an important ritual that is done by the father. Most tribal cultures still have one form or another that relates to this ancient ritual, but in our modern Western society, we often resort to books of names or simply a parent's middle name for our child.

In dreams, this ancient ritual, dormant in the conscious mind of fathers-to-be, is awakened by the knowledge that this man is about to become a father. For those future fathers who dreamed of being part of such a ritual and got a clear name for the child, it was an undeniably significant experience they took to heart. In most cases, the child was given the actual name the father-to-be had heard in his dream. Except for a few exceptions, this type of naming dream occurred mostly about the birth of boy children. The special connection between fathers and sons, the duty of the son to carry on the lineage and keep the family name alive, are rooted in ancient beliefs that probably reach deep into the dreaming life of future fathers.

The fathers-to-be all expressed a feeling of awe at being part of this ritual. For most of them it was an unforgettable story. It gave them a new perspective on the depth of dreams. In some cases, there was a new feeling of belonging to a greater community, a circle of fathers that was as old as time. For one father, his naming dream put him in touch with a part of his family history he had not even been aware of. For him, the dream took place in a Native American setting. Through it he reconnected with his own lineage, all the way back to his distant ancestors. After the child was born, he took the name from his father's dream, Cougar.

Cougar is a child who, just like his father, is fascinated with planes and helicopters. By the age of two, he could name the different parts of several planes and helicopters. Naming is also very important to Cougar. It is a habit of his to define his surroundings by discovering the proper name for the things he sees.

The mystical interaction of dream with reality (one

affecting the other) is not unusual where dreams of such visionary impact are concerned. These dreams are precious reminders that we embody a larger world than the one we know in our waking lives.

Whose Choice Is It, Anyway?

The act of making love with someone is an act of creation, whether we are creating intimacy, trust, emotional ties, or a child. This fact came home to Walter very poignantly when he was having intercourse with his partner. It was a completely new experience that utterly changed his outlook on parents and children, and made him question who actually does the choosing, the parent or the child. For Walter the experience was more disturbing than mystical. It shocked him into a new state of awareness, a new view of how life is created in the universe.

> *I am in the middle of making love to my partner, when suddenly I feel something behind me, a presence, a very powerful force, pushing my back. It is as if I am not in charge of this love-making anymore. Someone or something has its own agenda and is using me. I was overcome with this knowing right then, like an inescapable feeling, that I had created a child, or rather that a being had used me to enter into my partner's body. It was the most disturbing notion. It stayed with me for days. I tried to ignore it or dismiss it, but a part of me knew without any doubt that I had made her pregnant. When she*

walked into my office a month later, I knew she was going to tell me she was pregnant. I was right.

The most remarkable and disturbing part of the whole thing for Walter was his realization that there were greater forces than he had ever considered or imagined at work in the creation of a child. It made him feel unimportant, used by someone who needed his body to come into form. It was hard for him to believe that the act of making love was not just between him and his partner, but that there seemed to be other people involved, watching and waiting for the opportune moment to jump in, so to speak. It reminded him of an old Woody Allen film, where the sperms are getting ready to give up their lives for the next possibility of procreation, except in this case there seemed to be souls involved, not just sperms.

He started pondering the implications of this personal discovery and how a soul chooses its parents. He came to believe that it was not the parents' decision to have a child that was important but indeed the child's decision to come into form through certain parents that he/she had selected.

Soon Walter began to feel as if he had dreamed the whole thing. He started to believe it had been a figment of his imagination, an illusion. Even if what had come to him was a glimpse of the other side of life, it certainly did not fit his idea of a mystical experience. It was too uncomfortable to think about anymore so he put it in the back of his mind, where it kept nagging him once in a while like an annoying sound you cannot locate in your environment. But when his partner walked into his office a month after the event, she did not have to utter a word for Walter to know what he had been party to. He knew without any doubt that he was going to be a father. It was unbelievably clear.

The Forces of Change

In some instances, the unseen presence of his future child intrudes on the everyday reality of the father-to-be in a way that changes the person's life forever. This was the case for Reginald Gayle, who completely turned his life around after his baby boy was born.

Twenty-four years ago, Reginald was expecting his firstborn, his son Zaid. He had had a dream in which he had clearly seen his son and so had long decided on a male name. It was interesting to him, that although he was an atheist, the name he had chosen for his son meant something like "increase in the power of God." Reginald had a feeling that this child would change his life, but he did not know how or how much.

> *In the delivery room, I began to feel what I can only describe as "a sort of power surge," as if all the energy expended by everyone in the entire room, the doctor, nurses, my wife, was sucked into a spiral and went into her womb as she exerted her final thrust. I realized in that moment what the creation of our universe must have been like. This was the same thing on a human scale. It was the most extraordinary mir-*

acle. *I could have sworn there were other invisible beings in the room supporting this newborn baby and all of us. I had no frame of reference to put it in. But it was undeniable, tangible. I came out of that experience speechless. In my life it had the impact of an atomic bomb. I went from being a confirmed atheist to the realization that there was a God. Afterward, my whole life was rearranged. I no longer did any marijuana or drank alcohol. And almost immediately after Zaid was born, I began on a metaphysical path. I also became a vegetarian and I embarked on a more permanent career. The same radical change of life occurred in Zaid's godfather, who is still my best friend. It was as if my son had said as he came into the world," I am here now, and you better change your life, and prepare the way for me."*

This was the beginning of a completely new path for Reginald, a path that had begun with the mystical experience of his son's birth and continued with in-depth study of metaphysical subjects from Judeo-Christian beliefs to Buddism and African traditions. He chose the path of Religious Science, which was the most compatible with his spirit, as did Zaid's godfather, Michael.

A few short years later, he started to get recurring dreams in which a being he could not identify came to visit him several times. These dreams were filled with casual conversations, just like two people getting acquainted.

It was a pleasant conversation, but I also got the feeling I was being interviewed. We got along very well. We liked each other. It was very odd because it happened about four times in the space of a few weeks. Finally, she told me her name was Irisna. I remember chanting the name so I would not forget it when I woke up. I did not talk to anybody about this, not even my wife. It was a little unnerving.

The name of this female creature was stuck in his mind thanks to his chanting. For a reason he could not explain, it was important to Reginald to remember this name. He started thinking about having a second child, a girl, and calling her Irisna. Two months later he had another dream in which Irisna told him that she wanted to be born with him and his wife as her parents, if they were agreeable. Reginald said yes. He had no more dreams of her after that but told his wife about it. At the time she was on the Pill and had not been thinking about having any more children, but his dream struck a chord in her.

Six months later, Reginald had another dream in which three angelic-looking people came to tell him that now was the time for conception. Irisna was apparently ready to come into the world. Following the instruction of this latest dream, he told his wife to go off the Pill and two weeks later she became pregnant with the baby who would be their daughter Irisna.

By the time Irisna came into his dreams, Reginald was a practitioner in Religious Science, well entrenched on his new metaphysical path. It seemed natural to him to pay attention to the messages from his nightly stories and their visitor. The line between the world of the visible and the invisible was not as clear-cut or impenetrable as it once had been. The birth of his son had changed that forever.

Someone else might have ignored these visitations, thought of them as disturbances of the imagination brought on by stress or some other convenient pathological explanation. But the world in which the creation of new beings is first conceived of is in many ways still beyond the reach of our scientific minds. It is an irrational place, a place of heart, instinctual and ecstatic, and sometimes it comes to us through a glorious vision provided by our dreaming life.

To open yourself up to the visionary aspect of your life is not as strange or difficult as it sounds. You did it as a child with daydreaming. If you want to enhance this capacity in your psyche, make it more available in your daily life, you can try the exercise I provide for this purpose at the end of Part II.

The truth is, if you decide with a firm and clear intent that you want to be more open to the messages in your dreams and accept your ability to be an oracle in your own life, this will be enough to set the process in motion. The universe knows how to take a hint and make something of it. Take advantage of this time, while you are going through this pregnancy with your wife, to tune in to your dreams and recognize that they have the capacity to inspire and illuminate your life, past, present, and future. These men mentioned in the last chapter are ordinary men. I hope you understand both the ordinariness and the beauty of their psychic and visionary dreams.

• • •

Becoming a father is one of or maybe the most trans-formative event of a man's life. It opens the doors to a level of commitment to life that reveals itself in many different ways. This commitment first appears in dreams, working its way through the gates of the uncon-scious and rising until it reaches the conscious regions of the psyche. Whether full of anguish, exhilaration, or premonitions, these dreams are milestones along this path of transformation, helping a man cope with, understand, adjust to (and even foresee) his fatherhood.

As men and women, we are as similar as we are dif-ferent. Our fears and our dreams, our desire to love, be loved, be a good parent, is at bottom surprisingly iden-tical. Our capacity to dream and to have our dreams inform our daily life in a judicious manner is also not as dissimilar as we might assume, given the differences that have been emphasized throughout history and right up to this day.

So share your night stories with your wives. Dare to share your visions and your mystical dreams. You will find them receptive and eager to share their own wacky and tender dreams with you. Even if you remain skep-tical or dismiss it all, until all the hard facts are in, you will come to appreciate how exchanging such personal visions will increase your capacity for intimacy with your partner. You have nothing to lose.

Dreams are the language of the soul. They speak in metaphors, not in riddles. They are *your* metaphors, from your own mind. All you need to do is tell yourself that you will remember your dreams and that you will understand your language of the night. Tell yourself that you are willing to hear whatever information your soul has to offer you. Tell yourself that you want to find out more about what it means to be a father. Tell yourself that you want to meet your future child. Tell yourself that your dreams are your allies on this road to becoming a father. Give your psyche these instructions and in return your dreams will tell you who you are becoming, how you are changing or resisting change, and what it takes to become a father.

Dreams are your personal connection to the unseen, to the events that are yet to be. Dreams make an ideal partner in the realm of potential fatherhood or motherhood. They are humorous, thought-provoking, revealing, mind-blowing, challenging, sometimes soothing, and even reassuring—but the one thing you can count on is that they always carry more than meets the eye.

Believe in your nightly creations, trust your own feelings, and you will be amazed at the richness of information, guidance, and revelations that come into your life. More than at any other time in your life, while your wife is pregnant, it is important to be in touch with what makes you who you are. As a father it will help you parent your child with more understanding and patience for yourself as well as your newborn.

Between the fears and the yearning expressed in your dreams, here you are, poised on the brink of fatherhood, in some ways as naked and vulnerable as your newborn. Your dreams, like Hermes, the messenger of the gods, will bring new awareness, clarity, humor, and greater vision to your life. Armed with the wisdom of your dreams, you will be able to make a smoother, more conscious transition into the world of parenthood. If you start this journey at the beginning of the pregnancy, then you will truly have had the same nine months of preparation to enter this new phase of your life as your wife and baby.

A Final Note

The world of dreams closely resembles the world of the womb in which the baby is developing and learning to become a human being who possesses consciousness. In both environments—the womb and the dreaming space in the mind—infinite creativity, smooth darkness and the feeling of floating through timeless space, link like palms coming together in prayer. Through your dreams, you join the vast consciousness which is akin to the world of the universal mother your baby lives in as she is preparing for her birth. When you heed the messages of your unconscious, you are acknowledging the impact this new life is already having on your own development as a father-to-be.

PART IV

❧

The Basics of
Dream Interpretation

❧

However alien or foreign they seem, dreams are still the product of our own minds. Even though we may want to separate ourselves from the embarrassment of a sexual dream or the fear of a nightmare, we have no choice but to accept these night visions as the workings of our own soul. We are the dreamer dreaming landscapes worthy of a Jules Verne novel or a Dante poem; we are the creator of each fantastic event that fills our sleeping bodies.

Since many dreams are whimsical and abstract in nature, interpreting them requires an open mind and a receptive heart. Following are five methods of dream interpretation that should be a very helpful guideline. Remember, when it comes to analyzing your dreams, your first instinct is usually the best. When you observe a dream and an idea enters your mind, you should always trust it. Our souls move at lightning speed. When we are in tune with them we can analyze a dream in the flash of an eye.

If an image from a dream haunts you for days, let it. Even if the meaning escapes you at first, trust that it will be revealed in due course. A dream symbol stays with you because it has a significant message to impart to you. If you allow it to roam around in your conscious mind, sooner or later the key will appear and establish the link between the conscious and the unconscious part of the psyche. In that instant the revelation will present itself to you with unmitigated clarity.

CHAPTER TWELVE

Word Association

Word association is probably the most simple and straightforward method to interpret a dream. It works well with dreams that have recurring symbols or intriguing motifs that warrant your exploration. This is how it works.

To begin your word association interpretation you need to single out either a character from your dream or a meaningful object that appears to have some symbolic relevance. You then write the word down in the center of a page of blank paper and begin connecting other words to the main word as quickly and spontaneously as possible.

Here is a recent dream image in which a new type of mother energy is emerging. I will explain it to you and then do a brief word association exercise on the main character.

I am sitting in the kitchen of a large wooden house. There is an old woman with long dark hair and linen robes who is preparing food on the stove. She feeds me a delicious rib covered in sweet sauce, and then proceeds to give me a series of desserts made from fresh honey. When I finish eating, she touches me on the shoulder. I feel a gentle love rush through my being. She is like a mother. We have known each other before.

Now here is the word association based on the character of the old woman:

old woman-sweet-warm-tender-nurturing-skilled-observant-psychic-powerful-enchanting-hypnotic-intuitive-serendipitous-charming-loving-maternal-long hair-gentle hands

Once the list of word associations is done (and you can make it as long and varied as you are moved to), scroll down the page and let yourself absorb the impressions you have received. From this list, one senses that there is a new kind of mother energy present in the psyche of the dreamer. Great importance is now being given to nurturing, to food. Honey is the essence of food, in that it is pure, natural, and close to glucose, which is the primary nutrient of the body. The richness of the ribs covered in sauce on the other hand might be suggesting a need for protein. This might happen in the dream of a vegetarian or vegan. When she becomes pregnant, the mother-to-be might have dreams about eating meat or fish. She would do well, in that case, to take the necessary supplements to compensate for her dietary deficiencies.

You could of course stay with this very literal interpretation of the dream and find it satisfying. On the other hand, there is an obvious wisdom to the feminine aspect of the old woman character in the dream. She is informing the mother-to-be about the qualities she should value in herself and even the kinds of food to eat and lifestyle to lead. In other words, the old woman is suggesting a better type of environment for both the mother and the baby. The mother-to-be seems to be tuning into how to take better care of herself, to be more attentive to her emotional needs, and thus move closer to a balanced state of being.

In the list you make, words might appear that will surprise you. These are the words to watch out for. They are the ones that give you insight into what the dream really means. In the above list the words *powerful* and *enchanting* might be construed that way. It is not immediately obvious that an old woman could possess these character traits. The word association could be very enlightening in this respect for the mother-to-be. Through the exercise she may learn that her love is connected to a wise old woman archetype that is not weak, but rather nourishes the very foundation of her soul and is able to guide her at this crucial time.

In the dream, there were many more interesting images to draw from and use for a word association: like the rib covered in sweet sauce or the honey. This is how word association works. It lets you drill holes into the fabric of your dreams through which you may locate hidden jewels of information. Words have power. *The more we can define a dream linguistically, the more we can translate the abstract and whimsical details into useful fact.*

We are often scared of our unconscious because it is not familiar to us. We are afraid of what we will find there. The word association of the following dream shows how you can explore your unconscious in a way that is gentle yet penetrating. Here is the dream:

> *I am on a boat with friends. We are on the ocean. The weather is fair. The water is calm. A school of dolphins comes up to greet us. One of the females of the pack moves right to the side of the boat next to me. I see her dolphin smile on the side of her mouth. I reach out to greet her. She takes my hand in her mouth between her tiny teeth. She wants to pull me in. She wants me to join them, to come and play in the deep. I am not afraid.*

Here is the exercise from this dream. In this case, the idea of following the dolphin into the depths of the ocean was used as the basis for the word association. Rather than starting with a specific word or object, I started with the mental image of journeying under-water. The way to do this is to close your eyes and let yourself flow.

deep-dark-womb-feminine-love-maternal-offspring-laughter-dance-circles-infinity-life-blossom-tears-roots-liquid-love

In this word association, the acceptance of the dol-phin's invitation reveals a willingness to explore the maternal aspects of the woman's own nature. Instead of the foreboding unknown, when the dreamer breaks the surface of the ocean, there is a joyful recognition and a sense of coming home. The dolphin is in itself a profoundly feminine image, not just of the woman's unconscious, but truly symbolic of her emerging feminine wisdom as well as her nurturing ability. The fact that she has to dive in deep to find it has to do with the powerful transformation taking place in her body and in her emotional life as well. It takes courage to become a mother.

When you do this exercise, see if you can reconnect with the images and sensations of the dream by closing your eyes first and speaking the words out loud before you write them down. This is a great exercise to do in the later stages of pregnancy when your contact with the baby has become more defined. It will activate a dialogue between you and your child and allow for a deeper intimacy with your dreams.

Practice this word association exercise once a week and see how your dream interpretation improves. Soon the process will become second nature and you will be able to interpret dream images with an effortless flow. Trust your instincts and let your spontaneous mind lead the show.

CHAPTER THIRTEEN

Emotional Response

As dreamers we must be willing to identify our true feelings in the dream with as much honesty as possible. These feelings tend to mirror the feelings we have in our waking life with an impeccable accuracy. *In the dream state you cannot lie to yourself.* For instance, if in your waking life your relationship to your husband/ family/friends or co-workers is fine, but in your dreams you feel a great deal of frustration or anger toward this person, there might be something that you have not acknowledged about your relationship with her/him. Especially if the dream is recurring, then it is definitely a sign for you to explore the relationship on a deeper level and figure out what is causing the disturbance in your unconscious mind. During pregnancy, with hormones running wild, the emotional life tends to be even more "out there" and dreams will pick this up. It is actually much harder to lie to yourself or even be nice when what you truly feel like saying is, "I do not want anything to do with you right now."

The emotional palette of dreams is quite extensive: fear, bliss, anger, confusion, self-consciousness, embarrassment, anxiety, worry, sexual arousal, pleasure, pride, disappointment, unhappiness, contentment, peace, serenity, and much more. During your pregnancy, these emotions become more easily identifiable. Some might surprise you if you have not faced them in your waking life. But the dreams are here to help you clear out any unnecessary emotional burden so that you may concentrate on your relationship with your baby. This is not a time to be socially conventional or even gracious. This is a time to listen to the emotional truth and resonance of your dreams.

Finding the emotional tone of the dream as accurately as possible will help you not only interpret the dream, but also illuminate whatever situations are transpiring in your waking life. It will also assist you in living with less interference from your rational mind because the feelings we experience in our dreams are not tempered by our intellectual faculties. Every emotion happens with a kind of purity as when we were children. As dreamers we experience a freedom of movement from one emotional tone to another. For instance, in a dream we can go from the terror of falling to the bliss of flying in an instant. This is the magic of dreams. Each moment can be a new world, full of dynamic shifts and emotional impressions.

The following dream had a significant emotional content, with a healing effect on a particular relationship. I am providing this dream as an example of how you can interpret and integrate the emotional response of a dream into your waking life. This is especially relevant for the mother-to-be as her emotional life is more prominent at this time.

> *I am in a doctor's office alone in the waiting room. I am sitting in a comfortable chair. Although the atmosphere is cheery, I feel apprehensive. I have a feeling that whatever is wrong with me has to do with my feminine organs. As if to confirm that, my mother comes into the room (or at least I feel that it is my mother—but there is something different about this woman, something larger than life). She is the doctor. She stands behind me and puts her hands on my head. At first I don't trust her touch. Soon, however, I begin to feel a warmth emanating from her hands as they move over my entire body. The warmth is not only a sensation of light but becomes a powerful feeling of compassion and love that completely relaxes my body and opens my heart. It is almost overwhelming. I feel as if I am being healed by the mother principle of life itself. I wake up.*

In this dream, the dreamer experienced a kind of love much greater than she had ever felt in her waking life. You could call it a spiritual experience. Since it was her mother who was the vehicle for the love available in the dream, it forced her to look at her relationship with her in a new light. It also addressed some issues she had about her feminine body that might have interfered with her becoming pregnant and then accepting her pregnancy. The fact that the dream takes place in a doctor's office is very telling. The dreamer was worried about being able to get pregnant at the time. Thanks to the dream, she was able to accept the maternal principle as something real, something that had healing potential in her own life. Because the dreamer had allowed the imagery of the dream to live in her, it affected her waking life in a positive way.

This is how the emotional response interpretation works. You identify the feeling tone of the dream and then apply it to the relevant emotional situations in your waking life.

Try applying this technique whenever you have a dream that emotionally stirs you. It might lead you to resolve a relationship difficulty or a work-related conflict that could be affecting you in ways you have not anticipated, including your ability to deal with your pregnancy. It might also help you discover things about what you need and do not need at this sensitive period of your life. At all times follow your instincts. Stay in tune with your feelings and be honest about what is really going on in the dream.

CHAPTER FOURTEEN

Point of View

There is a common psychological theory that states that when we dream, each character and symbol we come across is in some way a reflection of ourselves. This means that if you have a dream of yourself being chased through the forest by a ravenous dog, not only are you the one being chased but you are also the dog. In other words, there is a part of you that is running from something and another part of you that is in pursuit. When we observe our dreams from this perspective, as a series of mirror images, we are more easily able to identify what type of conflict is going on within our psyche.

Most people are not familiar with this type of analysis. The average person does not want to admit that they possess any darkness. We always want to be the good person in the dream, the brave and noble one who is doing no harm. The truth is we are not made this way. On an energetic level, we are teeming with both positive and negative forces. When we accept this truth and begin to take responsibility for every facet of our dreaming life, from the darkest killer to the most radiant angel, then our waking life can become more balanced and the destructive tendencies that are being played out in our subconscious will be disarmed. This is very helpful for a mother-to-be because it gives her a chance to examine any kind of internal conflict she may have about her pregnancy, consciously or unconsciously, through the lens of the dream. The conflict can be addressed in the more archetypal context of the dream, which is in itself very useful and less threatening.

Here is an exercise you can perform to help you interpret dreams from this all-encompassing perspective:

1. Make a list of all the different characters and symbols in your dream.

2. Beside each character or symbol write down an adjective or series of adjectives that best represent the personality or idea that you have witnessed in your dream.

3. Briefly take on the role of each character or symbol and see how it relates to you personally. Remember, it is your mind that makes up the symbols and characters in a dream. In one way or another, they are all part of you. Even if they seem foreign, it is only on the surface.

4. Identify which elements of the dream you need to integrate into your waking life. For instance, if a character in your dream has a healthy expression of anger and you find this part of yourself repressed, you can

invoke their intensity into your daily life when it is appropriate.

Performing these steps will open your mind to the underlying tensions of the dream. You will begin to see yourself as a composite of forms, multifaceted and brimming with possibilities. Rather than defining the dream literally, the above directions will give you a chart that points out exactly what is going on beneath the surface of your conscious mind. You can follow this chart in several ways. For example, if a character in your dreams is dressed in sexually provocative clothing, you might want to take a second look at your maternity clothing and see if you can find something to wear that is comfortable and yet still attractive and sexy. A pregnant woman is usually vital, full of hormones that help brighten her eyes, make her hair shiny, her nails strong and long, her body limber. A pregnant woman can be very alluring, and a sexy dream could be reminding you that you indeed are sexy, sensual, and beautiful.

In this sense you are not only interpreting the dream but responding to it as well. You are absorbing the nutrition of the dream into your waking life much the same way a plant draws nutrients from the soil. The unconscious is dark and muddy. It is full of energy. When you draw something from your dreams into your conscious life, the dream lives on unwasted.

So the next time you have a dream look at it from all sides. Accept the fact that a part of you is living and breathing in each facet of the dream, from the drops of dew hanging on the forest branches to the white fangs of the dog that is biting at your heels. Not one detail in a dream is utilized in vain. Like a good painter, our unconscious mind is aware of every tiny stroke.

CHAPTER FIFTEEN

Metaphors

Most everything we see in a dream is a metaphor for something else. This is the way our unconscious speaks to us. It weaves together symbols and images into a metaphorical tapestry that we must decode in our waking life. Some of the metaphors we find in our dreams have a more literal interpretation and others are more abstract and imaginative.

I shall use the example of fire to illustrate this point. Say, for instance, you have a dream about a raging fire that is eating away at your house. In this case, the fire could be metaphorical for something in your life that is out of control. The dream might be trying to tell you that it is time for you to simplify your life so that you can attend to this pregnancy without feeling over-whelmed. However, if the fire is quiet and manageable, then it could be a metaphor for something else. It could be a metaphor for the feeling that you are creating with your new baby: the hearth of a home around which everyone gathers. It could be expressing your inner contentment with your own body, "on fire" with new life.

The metaphor will have different shades of meaning depending on how it is represented in your dreams. Common symbols such as a snake, a river, or a house can have a multitude of metaphorical meanings, and each requires an objective and detailed analysis.

Following is an exercise that will help you decode the metaphors that appear in your dreams. Use the guidelines but also listen to your own intuitive response. Sometimes a metaphor might be translated by instinct, with no logical steps whatsoever.

Read the rest of this section of the chapter and then try decoding a metaphor from one of your own dreams. Start with something simple and work your way up. Remember, all the metaphors in your dreams are produced by your own unconscious mind. No one knows what they mean better than you do.

EXERCISE

1. Choose a particular metaphor in a dream that has made a strong impression on you.

2. Examine the context in which the metaphor is set. (As I pointed out, a raging fire burning up a house is quite different from a quiet fire in a fireplace.)

3. List the natural or most commonly known proper-

ties of the metaphor. For instance, if you are attempting to decode the metaphor of a kitchen, list some adjectives that describe the average kitchen: warm, cheery, bright, and so on. (See Chapter Twelve, Word Association.)

4. Describe your relationship to the metaphor in the dream. Are you cooking in the kitchen or kneeling down? Are you happy or sad?

5. List your personal relationship to the metaphor in daily life. How do you feel about kitchens? Do you like them? Do you spend a lot of time in them?

6. Make an overall interpretation of the metaphor from the combined facts of the exercise.

The Dream:

> *I am standing in front of the stove. I am trying to get an apple pie to cook in the oven, but it just does not want to cook no matter how high I turn the fire in the oven. I feel very frustrated. I am getting upset at my ineptitude to cook this pie. Finally I just give up. Suddenly my cat appears. She starts to purr and jumps on top of the counter. She sits on top of the oven like a hen sits on an egg. I hear the fire start inside. The pie is finally cooking. I am so relieved. I thank her and walk out into my garden to sit by the little waterfall. That's all I really want to do, listen to the sound of the water and maybe read a little and rest. Through the open door I see my cat sitting on the oven, doing what she seems to know how to do, better than I—cooking. I wake up.*

1. The metaphor that I am going to interpret in this dream is the image of the cat sitting on top of the gas range. This cat obviously performed an important task for the dreamer.

2. The cat-by-the-stove metaphor has been around for a long time. It carries the feeling of home and comfort with it. This one is a little more unusual in that the cat is actually sitting on top of the stove. The cat also seems to be able to turn the stove on and be in charge of cooking the pie.

3. When I think of a cat on a stove, I think of the following characteristics: sensual, instinctual, relaxed, assured, comfortable, in charge.

4. In the dream, it is only when the dreamer gives up trying to cook the pie that the cat takes charge. The mood of the dreamer and the dream is transformed. From frustration the dream goes to a peaceful relaxed place, with the cat in charge and the dreamer actually walking out into the garden to listen to the waterfall.

5. Cats are an ancient and mystical symbol, from Egyptian mythology where they were regarded as sacred to their connection with the natural forces of life as the familiar of witches. Cats always seem to know something we do not. They can be enigmatic, always sensual, and very connected to the instinctual process of life.

6. In the dream, the apple pie is not really cooking in the oven until the cat takes over the process. This is beautifully clear. The dreamer cannot "make the pregnancy happen" through an act of will. It is clearly an instinctual, unconscious process, which is very well represented by the cat in the dream. What the dreamer realizes is that she needs to let go and trust the process. Pregnancy is not a logical, conscious event. It is the

process of life itself at its most mysterious. She needs to respect that and go to the "garden" outside her usual way of operating in the world in order to cultivate her ability to listen and be in the flow of life.

The metaphors that arrive in our dreams don't come out of nowhere. The reservoir of our unconscious is rich with images from childhood and early adulthood that have great resonance and meaning even if we haven't thought about them for years. So if a metaphor doesn't make sense to you immediately, look to your past for solutions. All metaphors have a point of origin. If you investigate hard enough, you are sure to find it.

CHAPTER SIXTEEN

Meditation

Meditation is a great tool to deepen your connection to your dreams. It can be used to interpret the hidden meanings of dream symbols that remain undefined in your waking life. Everyone has a different style of meditation. For dream analysis, it doesn't matter which style you use as long as you arrive at a place where you are quiet and relaxed. Mantras are often used in meditation to expedite this process, bringing the mind to a single point of focus. In the case of dream interpretation, the mantra that will be used is the mental image of the dream itself.

The point of this exercise is to relive selected material from your dreams in a conscious and objective way, hereby producing insights that you are not able to have when you are the dormant subject of the dream. Following are some simple steps to activate the meditation process for this method of dream analysis. If you happen to be a student of meditation already and have techniques for calming the mind that you are familiar with, then by all means use them. Meditation is the art of uniting the conscious and unconscious mind into a state of unified wholeness. You will assist this process by adding dream analysis to the equation. It will invoke a sense of relaxed clarity that will enhance your daily life.

1. Relaxing Mind and Body

• Environment—Our environment can greatly contribute to or disrupt a quiet state of mind. For this exercise, choose a place in your home that is free of external disturbances. Turn off the television, the phone, the radio. Disturbing sounds such as car horns, barking dogs, and other auditory intrusions can be subdued by using harmonious music or a small fountain with running water.

If you prefer being outside, you can choose a serene place in nature, by the ocean, under a tree, or in the desert—something that suits your personality. You might also want to give some thought to the fact that it is both you and your unborn child who are going to be meditating together, so the location should be one that is satisfying for both of you.

• Breath—There are many breathing techniques you can use for meditation. This particular one disperses anxiety and quiets the body quickly. Here's how it works: When you are ready to begin, take a very deep breath and hold it for a count of ten, visualizing the oxygen from the breath filling your bloodstream, every cell of your body, and feeding your baby at the same time. Then as you exhale naturally, consciously let go of all the toxins in your body. Also allow any anxiety or stress to drain from your mind so that the child growing inside of you may also be totally relaxed. Do this for both of you. Once you have completed this cycle three times, you are ready for the focusing part of the exercise. Continue to breathe as quietly and gently as possible from then on as you would do when you are sleeping.

2. Focusing the Mind

• Tools—The simple act of closing your eyes can sometimes be enough to focus the mind, but most of us need a little extra help. Staring at such articles as a candle, a mirror, or a photograph of a holy person or running prayer beads through your fingers can influence the mind to slow down and achieve its focus. In regular meditation, these techniques are used throughout one's sitting time, but in the case of this exercise, it is merely a point of departure, since the focus will soon be taken over by a dream symbol. You might also focus on something you have already chosen for your baby, like a mobile, a toy, or even a piece of clothing. This will make the meditation a very personal exercise, a way of tuning into life through your very own embodiment of its mystery.

• Positions—This exercise can last anywhere from ten minutes to an hour, so you should sit comfortably to accommodate your body size and physical condition. If you are in the later stages of pregnancy, it is probably best that you conduct this exercise in bed, propped up by firm pillows. As best as you can, try to keep your spine straight and relaxed. If you happen to be a person who leads with your head, remember to keep your chin down. This will keep your neck vertebrae in line with the rest of the spine.

It is not necessary for this exercise that you sit in a lotus pose or some other advanced position. This exercise is about dreams, not physical prowess. You are not in a Zen boot camp. Go for comfort. Select a position that enables you to remain alert and present in the moment.

• Prayer—Prayer is one of the most effective methods of focusing the mind. It brings the soul and the body into one harmonious unit, symbolized by the joining of hands. Prayer can be conducted in several ways. For this exercise, you can either invent a prayer to invoke the specific consciousness required for the interpretation of your dream or you can say a formal prayer that will align you with your inner spiritual forces. It is up to you.

Prayer is both an invocation and a benediction, guarding the intention with which you approach this work. It gives it a sacred container. Here is an example of a prayer you could say to focus your mind and prepare yourself for the final stage of this exercise:

Dear Spirit,
I ask you to open my soul
to the profound mystery of my dreams.

Give me insight and clarity
so that I may learn more about the relationship
between my sleeping and waking life
and be at one
with all parts of myself.
Thank you for the gift of dreams,
and so it is,
Amen.

3. Contemplating the Dream in Meditation

Once you have completed the above stages of meditation, you are now ready to bring the dream material into your awareness. This process is simple. Select a symbol or a series of images from one of your dreams and allow your mind to focus in with the same relaxed attention from the previous exercise. Just as if you were viewing a film, let the dream roll through your consciousness until you feel yourself crossing into the landscape of the dream. Let yourself become immersed in the dream until its reality becomes more vivid than your surroundings. From this vantage point, the interpretation will happen on its own. You will be attracted to certain moments of the dream and get flashes of meaning that will deepen your understanding. Let yourself be surprised. Expect the unexpected.

One of the images from a dream used for this particular exercise focused in on a dream character who was part woman, part mermaid. By contemplating the character in meditation, the detached perspective enabled the dreamer to view this disturbing image with equanimity. She realized that the mermaid part of the image represented her deep instinctual nature, coming from the depths and trying to integrate itself with the rest of her human self. The dreamer also felt as if she was being "pulled under" by the pregnancy itself. This sense of being waterlogged, common in the later stages of pregnancy, was present in the fish tail her body had taken on in the dream. In meditation, the need for integration became apparent. A way to speed up this process of integration was to consciously merge the two images in her mind's eye, to accept the underwater part of her pregnant feeling. To her own surprise, it also helped her get in touch with a different flowing lightness in her body. Accepting the deep-water nature of her pregnancy somehow helped her "lighten up." This is the beauty of the exercise. Not only does it help you interpret your dreams, it can also assist in psychological healing.

Meditation is just another tool to help you interpret your dreams. It is actually quite a natural experience that has been performed for thousands of years. Its healing properties on the mind and body are side benefits compared to the impact that it has on the soul. You can make meditation part of your daily routine or you can use it specifically to interpret a particularly daunting dream. Be patient with results. Meditation is a gradual process that deepens over time.

CHAPTER SEVENTEEN

Active Imagination

Another way to get insight into your dreams is through a process called active imagination. This is the most lively and entertaining method of dream interpretation and dates back to Carl Jung, who first coined the phrase. With active imagination you actually interview characters and symbols from the unconscious. The way this is done is quite straightforward.

To begin with, perform the first two steps of the meditation exercise to focus and relax your mind. Once you are ready, select a character or symbol from your dreams that you wish to interview. This could range from a killer chasing you through your house to a Chinese fan given to you by an empress. After interviewing many characters and symbols, I have found that even the foreboding ones have a specific contribution to make.

Once you have made your selection, view the character in your mind's eye and begin to ask it questions.

Start with basics, such as "Who are you?" and "What are you doing in my dreams?" and work your way to more personal questions. At first your mind will get in the way, intruding upon the interview with skeptical thoughts and harsh criticism. Just ignore it. After a while your intellect will give up and the interview will become more real.

To keep the dialogue flowing between you and the character, trust the first words that come through your consciousness and stay in the moment. If you censor what the character says to you or doubt the usefulness of its contribution, you will stall the process. Following is an example of an active imagination interview with a character from one of my dreams. I will list the dream first and then proceed with the interview. Remember, the person you are really interviewing is always yourself.

I am holding a little girl by the hand. We are in the forest. It is one of those fairy-tale forests, mysterious, magical, thick, lush. Light is streaming through the branches. We find our way to a clearing where a wooden cabin stands barely distinguishable from its surroundings. It is covered in green leaves and ivy. It is getting dark and colder, so we knock, but the door is half open. We walk in. There is a fire in the fireplace with a cauldron holding steaming liquid. As my eyes adjust to the darkness, I see a very large, very black woman squatting by the cauldron staring at me with a powerful yet loving gaze. She is smiling with one side of her mouth. She is wearing blood red robes and a dark green cape. I am mesmerized by her and a little scared.

*There are herbs hanging all around and glass jars
filled with odd ingredients like roots and mush-
rooms. The little girl is not afraid at all and
jumps on the woman's lap with a giggle of recognition. The woman stares at me. She says,
"Your little girl is safe with me. It's time that you
went out into the world and became the shaman
in your own life." I wake up.*

The old/wise woman is a very powerful archetype for
all women. When she appears in your dreams, it is a
good idea to spend some time getting to know her
better. She is definitely a character that can appear
during pregnancy. The wise woman also usually has
some interesting message to impart, which is why I am
choosing her to be the subject of this interview. I get
the feeling she actually wants to talk to me. She is also
articulate, entertaining, and physically interesting in
my dream, although the little girl is a close second. Not
only does she appear to possess great wisdom and
knowledge of the earth, but she also speaks with the
uncanny clarity of an oracle.

Q Who are you?
A I am the old crone, the wise woman, feminine power.
   I am the earth life of your body. I am your instinctual
   soul.
Q Why have you appeared in my dreams?
A Because you are ready.
Q Ready for what?
A Ready to let me take care of that little girl for you.
Q Who is the little girl?
A You know who she is, just as you knew who I am.

Q So the little girl is part of me?

A Yes, she is. She is ready to come home. I am the real mother, the one who can keep her safe and let her play.

Q What can I do in my waking life to feel closer to you?

A I am always with you: when you trust your intuition, follow your instincts, flow with the moment, when you love your body, when you take the time to breathe, to dance, to love. I am always with you.

Q Is there anything else I need to hear from you?

A I am the root of your life. Everything flows from this place. When you really know and understand this, you are free.

The extraordinary and somewhat mythical characters you will meet during these sessions are full of practical advice and common sense. They can assist you in your decision making, all the way from knowing when you should make a baby to how to handle the highs and lows of your pregnancy. The more you practice active imagination, the easier it will become to access its wisdom. At first it usually feels a little awkward to be talking with a dream character, but after a while the discomfort goes away and what is left is a wonderful inner dialogue that is both healing and full of discoveries. Use this exercise whenever you feel the need for a more immediate connection with your dreams. It will serve you well.

PART V

❧

Engaging Your Dreams

❧

The very act of placing a piece of paper beside your bed before you go to sleep with the intention of recording your dreams in the morning will increase your recall.

—*Dr. Gayle Delaney*

For most of us, dreams come in the night and then vanish by morning. We wake up with a vague recollection of images that are quickly swept away by our daily routines. Our conscious mind is never given the time it needs to absorb the gifts we have received during sleep. Either we find ourselves troubled by the unprocessed material of our dreams or we move through the day cut off from a vital aspect of ourselves.

This chapter will help solve these problems. It will discuss various methods for reconnecting with your dreaming life, thus enhancing the quality of your existence. If you have just recently become pregnant, this is an excellent chapter to read over a few times so that you can stimulate your dream recall and begin the exciting correspondence between you and your unborn child.

Remember, when you are pregnant, you are more connected to the mystery of life than at any other time. You are a channel for spiritual information. These following exercises should be easy to assimilate. Do the ones that come to you naturally and trust your intuition at all times.

CHAPTER EIGHTEEN

How to Remember
Your Dreams

Here are some practical things you can do to enhance your capacity to remember your dreams. Choose at least one or two that resonate with your soul. They will make a difference in the clarity of your recollection. After a short period of practice, your dream recall will improve significantly.

1. Paper and Pen

Keep a paper and pen near your bed at all times or, if you are into electronics, a small voice-activated cassette recorder. Doing this simple act will notify your unconscious that you are willing to participate in your dream life. You will start to remember your dreams more frequently.

If you are pregnant you might want to invest in a journal that will make it easy for you to document your dreams on a regular basis for the next nine months. Getting a journal with that specific intention is another clue to your unconscious that you are serious about remembering your dreams.

Having pen and paper or a journal to write in is also useful to set up a dialogue with your unconscious. Here is how it works: If you have worries concerning your pregnancy and/or decisions to make, write them down in your journal before you go to sleep. This simple act of writing down your thoughts, desires, or worries opens the door to your unconscious and gives it permission to come up with ideas or solutions during your dreamtime. Try it. It works.

2. Autosuggestion

For those of you who have a really hard time remembering your dreams, this is a very helpful exercise. Autosuggestion is a mild form of self-hypnosis. This is how it works: As you are lying in bed just before sleep, do the breathing exercise from Chapter Sixteen to focus your attention and then say to yourself three times in a low voice, "It will be easy for me to remember my dreams. It will be easy for me to remember my dreams. It will be easy for me to remember my dreams." Once you have finished saying this, stay lying on your back in a meditative state and repeat the breathing exercise until you drift into sleep.

You can also use this exercise in a more advanced

format in tandem with your journal writing. Once the writing is done and you have reached a certain clarity about what is bothering you, then you can use the information in the autosuggestion process. Instead of just telling yourself that you will remember your dreams, make up another sentence befitting the problem you seek a solution to. For example, if you are hesitating about which is the best cradle to buy for your baby, you could say the following: "My dream will show me exactly which is the best cradle for my baby." Or you can choose to keep the sentence more general: "My dream will tell me what the best solution is." You might also want to add something like: "When I wake up, I will remember clearly what solution my dream has offered me."

Keep the sentences short and simple and the directives to your unconscious as clear and concise as possible. Remember that whatever gifts your dreamlife offers you, you are free to accept or reject them. But take into consideration that these gifts were born out of your own mind, so try to glean their wisdom before you discard them.

3. Transition

The first moment of waking is extremely important for dream recall. It is in that transition time between sleeping and waking that the barrier between the conscious and unconscious mind is most easily traversed. So the minute you wake up, do not immediately start thinking about your day or jump madly out of bed. Give yourself some time to gather the images from the night. If your mind is a blank, just stay in bed for a few minutes and ask your soul for assistance. Then when you are ready, take your pen and paper and begin to write.

The magic of this time between waking and sleeping is wonderfully captured in the film *Ladyhawk*, starring Michelle Pfeiffer and Rutger Hauer. In it, the lovers are cursed to live one by day as a hawk and the other by night as a wolf. The only time they can catch a glimpse of each other is during the transition period between waking and sleeping or between night and day, when the sun and moon are both still in the sky. There is an inner enchantment that takes place between rest and wakefulness. It needs to be investigated with great care.

The following poem should give you a good idea of the scope and ramifications of this transition period in a way prose cannot. It is called, appropriately, *The Transitional Dreamer*:

> *I dream*
> *not bound by time or space*
> *sex or race*
> *not defined by age or color*
> *job or belief*
> *I dream*
>
> *Aware of the sleeping*
> *next to my waking*
> *I am transitional*
> *be quiet! wait!*
> *do not stir too much*
> *I'm in the elusive state*

How to Remember Your Dreams

which becomes illusion so quickly
in the waking world

I'm not back yet
I am still there
in the dreaming that stirs me
I am a woman or a man
an animal eating live birds
I close the door on myself
and open another one

I see a dancer in the dusty hall
through strings of light
helping a poet to his knees
praying with him
holding his forehead

I am an Indian dreamer
who knows the spirit of the elk
I am a Christian dreamer
who walked with Jesus
across the desert
I am the dreamer from the far east
who danced the Barhata Natyam
on the lotus flower

Shhh! do not wake me yet
I am a transitional dreamer
I am aware of my waking
I am gathering the particles of myself
I do not know if I will wake
with a cry or a smile
or if I will wake at all

I am aware of the sleeping
next to my waking
I am not quite here
I am transitional
I am stirring
I am collecting
I am gathering the riches
from my dreaming travels
so that I may remember
more of myself
than I knew before

4. Writing Down the Dream

There is something magical that happens when you begin to write down a dream even if you hardly remember a thing. The very act of placing a pen to paper stimulates dream recall. One image will lead you to the next and before you know it, you will have several paragraphs of writing. Remember, even if all you have is a feeling, jot it down. A feeling can evoke a multitude of images and memories. One feeling can take you down a path rich in discoveries you would never make if you did not take it. Even if all you remember is a vague symbol or part of a landscape or just the atmosphere of a dream, follow it like you would a stream back to its origin. If you take the dream image all the way to its natural resolution, it will be like draining a tall glass of cool, clear water on a hot and humid day. It will quench your thirst, revitalize you in a way that you would never expect a simple dream image to do.

As the days go on, your memory will become more specific and larger fragments of your dreams will come into focus. Just start writing and you will be amazed at what happens.

A final reminder: Give yourself permission to dream and then give yourself the time you need to remember.

CHAPTER NINETEEN

Identifying the Setting of a Dream

After you remember your dreams for a while, you will begin to realize that these nightly phenomena often have recurring settings. In this section we are going to show you ones most commonly found in the dreams of pregnant women and how to catalogue them in your dream journal. If there are any extra settings that I fail to mention be sure to include them in your daily recordings. I can only provide you with a general outline; your dreams are unique and personal to you and may require an adaptation of the following list.

Every dream has its own unique setting. In one dream you could be finding your way through a tropical forest with exotic birds and monkeys, and in another dream you could be trapped in your childhood home, eating dinner with all your least favorite relatives. Depending on what message your unconscious is trying to send you, the dream setting will vary a great deal.

Being able to interpret the setting of a dream helps you understand its meaning.

There are two basic types of settings we experience in our dreams: structures and landscapes. Structures involve any indoor setting, such as an office building or a church, and landscapes involve any outdoor setting, such as a meadow or a forest.

Your spatial relationship to the setting helps determine the interpretation of the dream. For example, if you are placed at a certain distance from a house as an observer, you might be admiring or longing for whatever the house represents in the dream. If, however, you are placed inside the house, then the house represents an integral part of your personality that is being shown to you.

Following is a list of the basic settings you will encounter in your dreams and the relation they have to your pregnancy. If there is a setting you come across that we fail to mention, let your intuition give you some assistance.

Houses

Houses are a common element in dreams. They often appear as a literal interpretation of our personality, our ego, or our body, in short, that which *houses* our spirit. Since our "house" is in a constant process of transformation during pregnancy it is not uncommon for it to show up quite regularly in dreams at different stages of the pregnancy. If in your dream you are viewing a house from a distance, it generally means that a part of you is longing for the security and stability that the house represents. On the same note, if the house you are viewing belongs to someone you know in your waking life, then it is likely that a part of you desires to possess certain qualities from that person's nature.

Another important factor is the size of the house and the material used in its construction. For instance, a big concrete bunker will evoke very different feelings from that of a wooden cabin in the forest. In early pregnancy dreams, a wooden cabin might indicate a desire to escape from the polluted civilized world and return to a more natural way of life, and a solid more permanent structure, such as the concrete bunker, might represent the fierce need to protect oneself from a hostile environment.

When the dreamer is placed inside a house, the interpretation shifts to encompass the personality of the one who is dreaming. Whatever is contained in the house becomes a reflection of the dreamer's daily life. For instance, a house could be filled with lots of friends and wild furniture or it could be barren and empty. The most important factor is how the dreamer relates on an emotional level to what is contained in the house. In the above example, there could be an actual need in the person's life to create more space for herself, or if the house is empty, it might indicate that she should allow more people and activities into her life. Again, it all depends on how the dreamer feels about the interior of the house. That feeling is the main criteria for interpretation.

Another thing to consider is the movement of the dreamer. Where he or she travels within the house is a reflection of what needs to be explored within the psyche of the person dreaming. For example, if the dreamer is going downstairs into the basement area, this symbolizes a need to become more familiar with the realm of the unconscious. If, on the other hand, the dreamer is climbing into the attic, this means there is a need for spiritual exploration.

The dreamer can also move from room to room within the house. This journey is symbolic of the various inner dimensions of the dreamer's personality. Very often in pregnancy-related dreams, a room heretofore unexplored will appear. The room might contain a crib or some other element that is related to the impending birth. In some pregnancy dreams, the dreamer may actually revisit a room from her own childhood and find in it various symbols relating to her own mother, thus tracing a full circle between generations.

To simplify the analysis of house-related dreams, here are a few questions you can ask. Where is the house standing? What is the house made of? Is anybody else in the house besides me? What rooms am I exploring in the house? Am I walking up or down the stairs? What particular objects attract my attention? How do I feel in the house? Am I content, happy, insecure, curious, peaceful, worried, angry?

Answering these questions will clarify your relationship to the house and give you insights into your personality. You will start to get an impression of what character traits are repressed in your psyche, what needs to be explored, what needs healing, and where you are at this time in your life. During pregnancy, such dreams take on a sense of urgency, as if the psyche was intent upon clearing the aspects of the personality that might interfere with the healthy development of mothering and fathering qualities in the future parents.

Churches

Dreams of churches are usually symbolic of a new spirituality that is awakening in the dreamer's life. Such dreams often appear at the onset of pregnancy, as if creating new life puts one in touch with the deep mysteries of life in a spiritual if not mystical way. The size and style of the church determine how this new belief system is breaking through into the dreamer's conscious mind. For instance, a dream of a wondrous cathedral laden with gold might symbolize that the dreamer has finally opened up to a set of values that will enable her to live abundantly, spiritually, if not necessarily materially. She will be providing a wonderful setting for her future child. On the other hand, a dream of an impoverished chapel could indicate that the dreamer's belief system is still one of poverty and self-sacrifice and it is time to address it now, before the child is born. Of course, the interpretation depends greatly on how the dreamer views each kind of church in his/her waking life, but in general, this is the way it goes.

Dreams of churches always express some sort of link with the divine. For this reason, around the time of conception it is very likely that a woman will have a dream of a church. She might even see a baby near the altar, lying in a crib, drenched in the sunlight pouring in through the stained glass windows.

Things to remember: If you are standing inside a church in your dream it probably means that you have arrived at a new level of spiritual awareness, whereas if you see a church in the distance and are unable to enter it, it most likely means that you are still searching for a new faith and will arrive at one soon.

Also, what you are doing in the church is important. If you are pacing around wildly with your hands in the air, it might mean that you are frustrated with God and are seeking a more evolved relationship with the creator. However, if you are kneeling peacefully in prayer and appear content and at ease, then it probably means that you are comfortable with your faith and will receive peace of mind in your daily life. During pregnancy, this type of dream shows that you are at peace with the process as well.

Again, here are some questions to ask yourself when you have a dream of a church. What religious faith does the church belong to? Is it a church, a mosque, a temple, a synagogue? Are elements from the more ancient Goddess religions creeping in, something that would address the feminine more directly? How do I feel in the church? What am I doing? Am I at peace? Am I nervous? How did I get inside the church?

While you answer these questions, allow yourself to enter a state of quiet meditation. Let the feeling of the church surround your body. Then ask yourself if this is the faith you want to live with. We often dream in the faith we were raised with as children. By the time we become adults, our faith has been sealed into our unconscious. Making the dream conscious is another way to bring our spirituality up to date. Remember, it is your choice. Your dream of the church is only a guideline. The type of spirituality you live with in your daily life is up to you. Ask yourself if this is how you want to raise your child. If the answer is yes, that is great. If the answer is no, ask your soul to guide you to your true faith with more dreams. And expect something real and wonderful to emerge.

Castles

Having a dream of a castle can mean many things. For one, it can mean victory. A castle can be symbolic of a battle you have won over such a thing as an illness or a difficult task. You could simply be feeling victorious because you got pregnant, and for you it was not easy and therefore feels like a real accomplishment. Dreaming of a castle can also mean that you are a self-protected person, that in order for you to feel safe in the world, you need to be surrounded by high walls, a moat, a drawbridge, and other castlelike structures. (If you are inside the castle, it has an especially symbolic reference to self-protection.)

During the later part of a pregnancy, a dream of a castle is a positive sign. It means that all is going according to plan, especially if there are bright-colored flags in the turrets. This is a definite indication that the baby is healthy and that the kingdom (i.e., your family) is eagerly awaiting his or her arrival.

If in your dream you are outside the castle, perhaps viewing it from a faraway path, then the castle usually symbolizes a set of goals that you are aiming for that might take months or years to fulfill. But if the castle is nearby, say, a few hundred yards from where you are standing, then it could indicate that your achievements will happen very soon.

Questions to ask yourself when you have a dream of a castle: Where am I in the castle—the king's bedroom, the kitchen, the dining hall, the dungeon? What type of castle is it? What state is it in? Is it in disrepair or in mint condition? What is it made of? For example, a castle made of glass will mean something entirely different than a castle made of gold or stone. Glass has its own properties, just as gold and stone do. Glass is transparent, clear, but also fragile. Gold, on the other hand, is the most precious metal, with magical properties, the subject of many legends and myths. Who is with me in the castle? Am I wearing modern clothes or ancient apparel?

After you answer these questions, close your eyes and visualize the castle in your mind. Is this a place you would like to live? If so, why? A dream of a castle can sometimes represent one's future destiny. Check your castle dreams every now and then and see if you are on track.

Forests

In most fairy tales and myths, forests are a powerful element in the story. They are part of the magical, often difficult obstacles the hero must surmount in order to reach his goal. In dreams, the same is true. Forests are the site of fears to be faced and treasures to be found.

When you have a dream of a forest, there is usually something in your instinctual life that lives hidden and must be recovered. For example, in the previous chapter we talked about the old shaman woman who lives at the center of the forest. Through the exercise we found out that she held the maternal awareness necessary to take care of the little girl. These are the types of characters we find in the forest, wise beings, gnomes, witches, individuals who are able to feed us rich information that can nourish our lives.

If you dream of a forest while you are pregnant, it is especially important to identify the specific messages and symbols shown to you as you walk through the trees as they could be part of your initiation into motherhood: a gold ring, a chalice, a strand of pearls. Many precious treasures can be found in the forest, some of which are symbols of fertility. Go back into your forest dream and try to remember everything that was shown to you. Most likely the objects you find will offer you guidance for your pregnancy, even how to perceive and handle its ups and downs. During pregnancy, a forest dream might also be addressing a deep need to connect with and be attuned to this specific aspect of Mother Nature. This is an opportunity for you to realize that this important connection might be lacking in your waking life.

Here are some questions to ask yourself when you have a dream about a forest: What type of forest is it? Is it ominous or friendly? How do I feel walking through the forest: scared, curious, worried, lost, in awe? Is there anyone else in the forest? Are the trees able to talk to me? What animals cross my path? Are they dangerous or friendly? Does anything catch my attention? Is there a river I need to cross?

While you answer these questions, picture yourself immersed in the forest listening to the sounds of nature. See if you can get a general impression of what the forest is trying to tell you. Open your mind and soul to the beauty of your dream. What do you hear? What is the forest saying?

Mountains

Dreams of mountains are generally a fortuitous sign. They symbolize the various stages of a journey that the soul is undergoing on its path to wholeness, and pregnancy is definitely a great journey. Most dreams of mountains include some sort of climbing expedition or radical ascension. The dreamer could be scaling the mountain with his/her bare hands or flying up to the top of the peak with silver wings. Where the dreamer is situated on the mountain gives great insight into the meaning of the dream. For instance, if the dreamer is at the middle point of the mountain, and making steady progress upward, it would indicate that some under-taking (like a pregnancy) is well on its way to comple-tion. If the dreamer is at the bottom of the mountain, then the project or baby is still in "embryonic" form and might take a while to arrive at completion. Inversely, if the dreamer is at the top of the mountain, this would symbolize that something concrete has been accom-plished and the baby is now ready to be born.

The dreamer might also be climbing down the mountain. This often means that there has been a let-ting go or surrender of some kind. The onset of labor could be close at hand. Also, if the dreamer is traveling down the mountain it means that he or she is ready to leave the lofty heights and come back to earth in some way. In short, the need for separateness has been replaced with the need to belong, which the prospect of motherhood could very well symbolize for the dreamer.

Mountains can also have a literal meaning in our dreams. They can tell us simply that we need to spend more time outdoors, that we should let go of our city habits for a while and have an adventure in the wild. Pregnancy, after all, is a *wild* experience, and the outdoors are a natural setting for Mother Nature in all its manifestations. Mountain dreams can also be a symbol of great health and endurance, telling us that we are in *peak* physical condition, ready to take on the challenges of our life, an especially good omen for your pregnancy. If you have had any doubts about your physical health, this type of dream should relieve your fears.

Here are some questions to ask yourself when you have a dream with mountains in it: What kind of mountain is it? Is it familiar? What season is it, winter or summer? What is the weather like, sun, clouds, rain? Am I going up or down the mountain? Am I tired or exhilarated? Are there other people or animals on the mountain or am I alone? Are there any streams or lakes on the mountain? Do I feel at home or like a stranger?

While you answer these questions, hold an image of the mountain in your mind's eye. Let it speak to you on an intimate level. There might be some message or idea that you are supposed to receive. Mountains are a gateway to higher thinking. The symbol of the mountain from your dreams can open your mind to new vistas, leading you to think thoughts of a higher order. They are a reminder that pregnancy is a way to a new reality. And both father and mother-to-be often start thinking about the world and their place in it in a different way once they know that they are bringing a new being into it. The priorities can change from "got to get the latest cell phone" to "what can I do to make the world a safer, more beautiful place for my child." Mountain dreams can be a call to thinking differently than you have until now because this new being you are entirely responsible for is involved.

Meadows

Meadows (especially when they are filled with flowers) are a symbol of spring and renewal. The open space is not threatening like a dark forest but, rather, inviting, beckoning you to stop and lie down or have a picnic. Meadow dreams that invoke such feelings of relaxation and peace often occur in prepregnancy when a woman is beginning to consider the mothering aspects of her personality. In a dream, one young woman witnessed the transformation of a desert into a meadow. The earth went from being barren and devoid of all life to a field of flowers and fruit trees with birds and wild animals. In this case the pregnancy was a powerful transformative agent. A meadow filled with spring flowers could also indicate that the baby's arrival is very much a joyful event, appreciated and anticipated with happiness by the parents.

The presence of water, such as a river or a lake, in the meadow is a confirmation that fertility and motherhood are indeed the themes of the dream. Think of the waters of the river Nile in ancient Egypt fertilizing the valley and assisting in crop development. Water brings new life; it is a symbol of growth and change. Even in the middle of a winter scene, if water begins to flow, it is a sign that there is a thawing out, that Nature is coming back to life.

Here are a few questions that can help you interpret

the meaning of a meadow dream: What kind of meadow is it? What elements does it contain? Is anything missing? Where am I in relation to the meadow? Am I looking at it from a distance or am I standing in it? What am I doing in the meadow? Am I relaxing, strolling, hurrying? Is there something unusual about the meadow? What is the weather like; is it spring, summer, or winter? Does something catch my attention? How do I feel, happy, anxious, surprised?

This is *your* dream. When you review it in your mind, do not judge it. Be objective. This attitude will help you gather the information from the dream in greater detail. Be as open as the meadow itself and you will receive rich answers. The most important thing is to pay attention to the kinds of feelings the dream evokes in you. If you are already pregnant, the dream could simply be a reflection of your own blossoming, of the new life growing inside of you.

Caves

A woman who dreams of caves while pregnant is very involved with the process of her own pregnancy. She really knows what it means to be a vessel for the creation of life. She recognizes that she is an intricate part of the mystery and miracle of creation.

Cave dreams are particularly interesting because they can represent both a man-made structure or a natural setting, one that often includes rocks and water. Caves are generally believed to symbolize protection, a haven from society, and also represent feminine sexuality.

During the various stages of pregnancy, it is not unusual for an expectant mother to have recurring cave dreams as they are a powerful symbol of Mother Nature and the womb. Because of the onslaught of "raging hormones" in the first trimester (when the body is striving to keep up with the creation of a new life), the cave can often be invaded by ocean waves or wind. In this case, the cave dream expresses perfectly what the feminine body is going through at a cellular level.

In the second trimester, when, in most cases, mother and baby have settled into a more harmonious rhythm, the cave dreams will also reflect the dreamer's relationship with Nature. For instance, there could be a feeling of having to surrender to the awesome powers at work so that mother and child may become one with the process of creation.

The second trimester is a time when the mother deepens her connection with her feminine nature. During this time, the cave could be portrayed as a real haven, a retreat. The dreamer might be painting or decorating the cave, as was done in prehistoric times. This activity reflects a woman's need to create a nest, a safe place for herself and her baby.

In the last trimester, cave dreams might express a feeling of confinement or in other cases symbolize "a light at the end of the tunnel." Birth itself is an awesome event, bigger than our human minds can comprehend. The cave dream can show in what state of mind the mother-to-be is, whether she is willing to "ride the wave" or if she has a lot of resistance. The cave dream will even help determine where the resistance is coming from and why.

Cave dreams can be extremely useful. They can be a

source of guidance for a woman on the verge of giving birth. Here are some questions to help you interpret cave dreams: What type of cave is it? What does it look like? Is it dark or is there an opening through which light or water comes in? How do I feel in it, at ease, anxious, terrified, overwhelmed, peaceful, excited? Are there any intrusions? How does this affect me? Are there other men or women with me? If so, what are they doing and how do I relate to them? Am I alone? Is anything else going on? Am I involved in an activity? Do my feelings change during the dream?

CHAPTER TWENTY

Identifying the Theme of a Dream

Although each dream we receive is a unique expression of our soul, there are common universal themes that cross the boundaries of nationality and social background. Following is a cross section of the most common dream themes, ones that most of us have experienced at least once in our lives whether we are pregnant or not.

Pregnancy gives the dream a particular "reading," a slant, if you will, that we will explore in the chapter, but these themes can also occur when you are not pregnant. As you are reading through the list, write down any of your own dreams that fall into similar categories. Remember, as human beings we are all linked by our daily interaction with the world and this is reflected in our dreams. Do not be surprised if your memory is stirred by this study of themes. The dreaming world has touched us all in similar ways.

Colors

Whether we are aware of it or not, color is always present in our dreams. If we remember a particular color after we have awakened, it usually means that it has some significance and we would benefit from its examination. How we respond to a color in our dreams determines its meaning. For instance, red can mean danger or warning, but if we feel joyful in its presence, then it can symbolize creativity, vitality, and new life.

Another criterion in determining what a color means is the specific quality of the color: whether it is bright or dull, muddy or clear. If you look at the color yellow in your dream, its degree of brightness or dullness will help you uncover its meaning. In various Eastern religions, the color yellow is associated with the light of life itself and with health. A muddy yellow is associated with betrayal, faithlessness, and a lack of courage. The more you know about a color and what it symbolizes, the better you will be able to interpret its presence in your dreams.

Sometimes the easiest way to interpret a color is to associate it with other symbols. For instance, the color green could be associated with the basic color of Nature itself. A lush green could be a reminder of abundance, even paradise. The color blue often symbolizes spirituality. In Christian religions, it specifically relates to the Virgin Mary. For this reason, women who are pregnant might have a lot of dreams with blue as the dominant color: blue sky, blue ocean, blue clothes. They might feel as though they are carrying something holy, a Christ child of their own.

By the same token, the color white may be seen as a

pregnancy color; white expresses a link to the spirit world, the place from which all new life emerges. Though black is not a color, it is a very powerful symbol. Not only does it symbolize death and the void, but it also represents a state of surrender that we must come to in order for a new universe to be born.

Different colors may correspond to different stages of pregnancy: from white and blue in the beginning of the pregnancy, to the fullness of green or bright yellow in the second trimester, and finally red and even black as the mother comes closer to giving birth. Red in this case is being associated with the fire of creation, of life itself, and the energy of labor, of giving birth. Black is associated with the unknown, the "leap of faith" necessary for any endeavor, particularly for the quality of *surrender* required from a woman as she is about to enter the birth process.

Here are some questions to ask yourself when you have a recurring color in your dreams: How bright is the color? Is it muddy or clear, rich or pale? What does the color remind me of? How does it make me feel?

As you answer these questions, take yourself into a quiet meditation and let the color fill you up from your head to your toes. Let it guide you to a clear interpretation. Let go. Don't hinder its message.

Flying

Like any dream theme, flying can mean many things. In general, it refers to freedom and release. When we have a flying dream, more often than not our subconscious is telling us that we are in fine working order, that our psyche is well balanced and new opportunities are lurking on the horizon. Of course it is important to check with your own feelings in the dream.

For a pregnant woman, having a flying dream is a fortuitous sign. It means that she and the child have entered a spiritual relationship and are able to interact with each other in a shared weightless environment. If the flying dream comes in the later stages of pregnancy, it generally means that the mother will have an easy birth. The delivery will be buoyant and full of ease.

Here are some questions to ask yourself if you happen to have a flying dream: Where am I flying? What is beneath me? How do I fly, with wings, a glider, a flying machine? How much control do I have over my flight? Where am I going? Where will I land?

As you are answering these questions, go back in your mind to the dream scene and feel in your body the same joy of flight you felt when you were asleep. If you are pregnant, take this feeling with you into your day. Move with it, dance with it. Let the feeling of flight guide you in your waking life.

Pursuit

During pregnancy, a dream of pursuit could mean that the dreamer is afraid she is no longer in control of her life or her body. Nature has taken over. The instinctual world has flooded her unconscious mind, leaving her with a momentary feeling of helplessness. The father, too, can experience these types of dreams. Knowing that his own life is undergoing a deep transformation, the father can receive vivid images during sleep of being pursued or even trapped by wild animals, monsters, or savage people. These dreams, of course, are not harbingers of misfortune. They are a natural part of the process that every human goes through on the path to becoming a parent. They are wired into us, as ordinary as our patterns of waking and sleeping.

Here are some questions to ask yourself when you have a dream of pursuit: Am I the one who is being chased or am I the one chasing? Who is the pursuer? Do I know them? Are they from this world? Is it a dangerous animal or is the animal kind? How do I feel about this character? Am I terrified or amused? Is it a game or a life-and-death situation? How do I handle the chase?

As you are answering these questions, go back into your dream and see if at any point in the chase you turn to face the pursuer. In other words, is there a time when you stop running? If so, this is a good indication that you are taking a stand in your waking life and facing up to the issues that need to be worked out. If not, go over the dream in your mind and imagine yourself stopping and facing your pursuer. What do you think would happen? What would you discover about your pursuer, about yourself? Try it as an exercise and watch out for the revelations.

Eating

Sometimes dreams of food and drink are simply related to our physiological condition. During pregnancy, eating becomes extremely important because "you are eating for two." In other words you are feeding someone else besides yourself, someone who needs the food to create itself with. Your dreams in this case could be pointing to some specific food you need more of in your diet. Your unconscious might be telling you, "You need to eat strawberries" or "You need to drink more water," and consequently your dreams will be filled with these images.

Food dreams can also be related to spirituality. If you, for instance, dream of bread and wine—which are part of the typical sacrament used in many religious rituals—this might be a message from your unconscious that this time of pregnancy is pulling you toward a more spiritual view of life. The same would be true if you dreamed of eating fresh fruits from a tree. This could be symbolic of a need to have a closer connection with your spiritual nature.

Dreams of food and drink can also have a sexual dimension. The most obvious one would be eating a banana or a tomato, both of which symbolize the fecundity and pleasure of sex. Sexuality is part of a woman's life, especially when she is pregnant. After all, pregnancy is the very embodiment of what sex is about, creation. Also, with the hormones at an all-time high, a pregnant woman can feel particularly sensual and sexy, at least during the first half of her pregnancy, if not at the end of it. On the other hand, a dream of food and drink might be referring to the way the pregnant woman is relating to her pregnancy. How she eats the food will be indicative of her state of mind. If she is picking at it, the dream might show that she is not quite ready to be a mother yet. But if she is eating with a healthy appetite, the dream would mean that she has come to a place of acceptance and is nourishing herself for the upcoming demands of motherhood.

Following are questions you can ask yourself when you have a food-related dream: Am I longing for the food or does it repulse me? Is it freely available or do I have to work for it? What am I eating? Do I like it? Is it furfilling or does it leave me empty and wanting more? How am I eating, with gusto or am I picking at the food? Am I eating with utensils or my bare hands? How do I feel about eating this food? Is there guilt involved or is the eating a delicious experience?

As you ask these questions, close your eyes and remember the taste and texture and color of the food. Let the sensations move freely in your body. Imagine you and your baby being nourished on the deepest level. When you eat your next meal, bring this new awareness with you to the table. Make eating a sacred exercise. Remember, food is very much connected to love.

Nudity

Many expressions in our language refer to a state of disclosure. We are confronted with the "naked truth" or the "bare facts." Dreams in which we find ourselves naked or with minimal clothing can be pointing to a situation in our life (or an aspect of our personality) with which we are not comfortable. A dream that includes nudity might be trying to bring out the "naked truth" about how we really feel about something. The context of the dream is, as usual, crucial to its interpretation, as well as the feelings the dream exerts upon the one dreaming.

When a pregnant woman has a dream in which she is naked, it often refers to the profound sense of vulnerability she feels while carrying her baby. If she is well along into her second trimester, it could also mean that she finds herself at the center of a lot of attention with nowhere to hide. Her being "big with child" is increasingly visible to the naked eye. A nakedness dream could also indicate that a woman is feeling physically or sexually unattractive to her partner. In such a case, the crowd that surrounds her in the dream might appear repulsed by her nakedness. All these are clues to your inner state of mind and can help you and your partner navigate the waters of pregnancy more easily.

During the pregnancy, the father might also have nudity dreams that reflect *his* vulnerable state of being. And he can also have dreams that signify the exact opposite. One man had a dream in which his sexual organ was prominently displayed to a cheering crowd. The dream indicated that he was not feeling vulnerable at all but rather very proud of his potency, his ability to plant his seed and engender life.

The following questions will serve you well if you are trying to interpret a dream where your nudity plays a central part: Where is this dream taking place? Am I alone or is there a crowd? How is this crowd acting or reacting? Do they notice me or are they indifferent? Are they jeering or applauding? Do I feel vulnerable, scared, or confident? Am I comfortable or trying to hide? How do I feel?

As always, your feelings in the dream are the best

clues and should be examined closely with as much honesty as possible. When you review the dream, do not judge it, but, rather, become part of it again; let it unfold like a movie and catch each moment and its particular atmosphere. Remember you are the writer, actor, and director of your own dream. Be a detective. Explore the gifts your soul has laid bare for you. Dreams can sometimes be full of humor. You might discover an element of your personality you did not know you possessed until now.

Sex

As with nudity dreams, when you are interpreting a sexual dream, the context is very important. For instance, if you are alone, exploring your own sexuality, the meaning of the dream will be quite different than if you are having sex with another person or making love in a crowd with onlookers and other participants.

Dreams where sexuality is prominent are a signal to the dreamer that something needs attention in their sexual persona. It could also mean that the dreamer's libido has been repressed in some way and wants to be attended to. In other words, you could be needing more sex in your life. If you are pregnant, you might have to talk to your partner, let him know it's okay to have sex even if you are pregnant. Talk with your doctor about it if need be.

Sexuality is a very powerful creative energy. In many Eastern religions it is thought to be connected to life itself, to transformation, and to the cycles of death and rebirth. Because of this, dreams of sexuality can shed light on your feelings about life and death as well as your beliefs about immortality. This is especially true for women who are pregnant. A sexual dream for a pregnant woman can signify a celebration of life, a joyous acceptance of the part she plays in the cycles of death and rebirth. After all, when you have a baby, a part of you lives on. You create a biological chain of energy that survives the onslaught of time.

In most sexual dreams, there is actually very little sex. It has usually more to do with touch and desire than with the sex act itself. However, there are some exceptions. In one particular dream a woman found herself making love to what she called "a Christ-like figure." It was a very powerful dream for her. She was, in her own words, "making love with God." In this case the sexuality was an expression of her own deep-seated spirituality at this time in her life. She was simply embracing her own soul in a very physical, real way. God was not a heavenly figure somewhere in the clouds but part of the most basic and natural fabric of her life. The dream left her feeling renewed with a faith and trust in life she had never experienced before. Her pregnancy went on with an ease that she had not felt beforehand.

There are many types of sexual dreams, all of them reflecting an inner tension between our conscious and unconscious minds. A sex dream is an opportunity to integrate, to heal something that has been buried, denied, or sometimes longed for. It is not uncommon to have such dreams during pregnancy as your whole self is involved in creating this new life and wants the clearest, most whole environment for it to be born into. Since essentially you are this environment, your dreams endeavor to provide a ground for the healing of unresolved issues. Such dreams can also reflect a desire to feel more powerful in your waking life or they can put you face to face with your feelings of powerlessness. It confronts you with your true feelings about being pregnant, becoming a mother, and whether you are as happy as you believe you are about it. It is important to make these feelings conscious without judging them. Otherwise they will affect your pregnancy and your baby unconsciously.

Here are some questions to help you decipher the meaning of a sexual dream: Where am I? Am I an onlooker or a participant? Am I alone or with someone else? Who are they? How do I feel about them, interested and excited or repelled and embarrassed? Am I frightened or indifferent? Do I feel powerful or powerless? Am I in control? What is the overall feeling of the dream? Does it have a dreamy quality? Is it crude, animalistic, or romantic? What is it telling me about myself? Is anything surprising and why?

When you go over such a dream, put yourself in a receptive state. Relax. Be your own best friend. Let go of any moral judgment. All dreams are deeply connected to life, be it mental or physical. Dreams are not bound by morality; they live on a higher spiritual plane and embrace all experiences. Dreams render life like master painters or filmmakers. Let your dreams inform you, teach you, and help you understand yourself better.

Travel

It is quite natural in our dreams to travel to faraway places that we have never visited in our waking life. We might take a bus along some old mountain road to a primitive village far from the reaches of civilization. Or we might end up in some Alice-in-Wonderland kind of setting, with animals that speak and trees that know our name. Whatever the case may be, travel dreams tend to include a lot magic and mystery. For the most part, they signify change and advancement on your spiritual path. Pregnancy can feel like "traveling to a foreign land" in many ways, and travel dreams clearly express that feeling.

When you dream of a foreign place, it means that you have arrived at a new point of consciousness in your daily life. It acknowledges that, as a pregnant mother-to-be, you are indeed a different person. Your attitude has shifted to incorporate new physiological and philosophical perspectives. Your old ways of being are now outdated. It is time to see the world with fresh eyes and behave as though you have just been born because as your baby is being born, so are you, into motherhood.

An important thing to observe in a travel dream is the type of world you are visiting. What are the customs, the habits, the specific laws of the natives? By identifying these particulars, you will receive a clear idea of what type of energy your pregnancy holds for you and how it is affecting your life. For example, if the land you visited in your dreams was full of celebration and excitement, then it is likely that in your waking life you find pregnancy brings you a renewed joy for living, that it is full of rich spontaneous experiences leading you on your soul's path.

If you are not pregnant yet, a travel dream can give clues of things to come. Travel dreams are sometimes the way the soul prepares us for crucial changes in our lives. They can set the stage for what is about to happen, showing you the ways in which you need to expand your mind and how you see the world.

In travel dreams, your mode of transportation is just as significant as your destination. Driving a beat-up truck would have a different meaning than cruising through the air in a streamlined jet. If you are a person who is always speeding through life, now that you are pregnant, your dreamlife might be telling you to slow down with dreams that have you loping along in a horse-drawn carriage or walking barefoot through the forest. Examine your mode of transport and see how it relates to your waking life. Remember, as humans we are always in movement. Even the most homebound of pregnant women who has to stay in bed for days on end is still partaking in the most amazing journey, where every day, sometimes every hour, is almost like a new country.

Here are some questions to ask yourself when you encounter a travel dream: Where am I? What is the name of the land I am in? Do I relate to the natives? Can I speak their language? How did I get here? Did I drive, sail, run, fly? What is the purpose of my visit? Am I free to leave or am I stuck here for good? What is my favorite thing about this world? Is there something like it in my waking life? If so, how are they different?

When you answer these questions, close your eyes and visualize the world you have visited. Is this a place you would like to live? How can you make your daily life more in tune with your travel dream? If you are pregnant, see you and your baby existing in this world together. If it makes you feel happy, go there in your meditations whenever you are feeling out of sorts with the world around you. Let your soul lead you home, take you to rest in a land that is at one with your heart.

CHAPTER TWENTY-ONE

How to Empower Your Dreams

As dreamers we tell ourselves impassioned, strange, ghoulish, exhilarating stories. Sometimes we wake ourselves up because the dream is just too overwhelming and other times the outside world wakes us up before the dream is finished, with a phone call or the beep of an alarm clock. In such cases, many of us experience the desire to go back and complete our dreams. This takes an intense amount of concentration and of course luck. We are not always fortunate enough to reenter a dreaming sequence in the place that we left off. If this is the case, a successful method of finishing your dreams is to use your imagination to complete the ending. This is a very effective tool for bridging the gap between your conscious and unconscious mind. It is also a very healing practice, sending a signal to your psyche that you are willing to participate actively in all the dreams that your waking life inspires.

Following is a list of techniques you can use to empower your dreams, giving them the extra dimensions that you failed to accomplish in your sleeping state. Try each one and see what works best for you. Remember, your imagination and your unconscious are deeply connected. The dream endings you make up will not appear merely by chance. They will have their own psychological meaning, more real than you would ever imagine.

Fantasy

When you wake up in the middle of a dream, spend five or ten minutes lying in bed fantasizing about the ending. The transitional state between sleeping and waking is charged with creative energy. Use these forces to penetrate deep into your imagination to uncover a conclusion for the dream that gives you a feeling of satisfaction and ease. If you are pregnant, place both of your hands on your stomach and feel you and your child working through the dream together. If it was a nightmare that you awoke from, find some way to wrap it up that gives you peace of mind. Seek out the light in the dream. Use it to your advantage.

When you are doing this exercise, don't censor yourself at all. If your mind presents you with a series of wacky endings, enjoy it for all it's worth. Who knows, maybe one of them will turn into a movie script or a short story. Dreams are great fuel for creative projects. Many of the great works of art in the world found their genesis in sleep. Be open to whatever wants to come to you. And most of all, have fun.

Writing

After you have given yourself adequate time to fantasize about an ending to your dream, pick up a pen and paper and begin to write it down. This will help you reap the wisdom of the dream world for your waking life. With the writing will come a feeling of reality and acceptance, often accompanied by new insights.

Following the writing of the dream itself you might want to jot down how the dream made you feel and why it was important for you to complete the dream or change its ending. Such was the case with a dream of a woman who came to me for an interview. Her dream went something like this:

> *I am driving in my car, which is painted with a multitude of different patterns. I am driving along the highway quite fast when I see a small white animal on the side of the road. I try to avoid it, but I hit it instead. I can't believe it. I am devastated. I stop and get out of the car. It's a beautiful white little puppy. It is lying on the road lifeless. I cannot bear it. I have to do something. I have to bring it back to life. Somehow that is essential. I wake up.*

The woman awoke from her dream crying. She felt that the puppy was very precious and that her carelessness had killed it. She couldn't bear the thought of this, even though it was just a dream. She tried to calm herself down by closing her eyes and visualizing the scene. Instantly, a new ending for the dream entered her consciousness. She saw herself bending over the puppy, breathing life into its frail body. There were a series of witnesses standing around her, but she didn't let them distract her. She continued to blow into the puppy's mouth several times until finally the puppy came back to life.

Writing about the experience afterward, the woman said that imagining a new ending for the dream gave her great peace of mind and revealed important information about her own life. Doing a word association writing exercise, she realized that the puppy in the dream symbolized the most precious part of herself— her instinctual nature—and that she had almost sacrificed it by speeding along in her car. She discovered that if she didn't stop to take care of her inner self, she might become an empty shell, one of those people who identifies more with what they do in the world rather than who they are as human beings. Imagining a new ending for the dream, she said, was the first step in reclaiming her animal nature, the sacred part of herself that was in tune with the earth and the cycles of life. This seemed particularly relevant and poignant because she had just become pregnant and the dream was speaking to her loud and clear. This was the time to reevaluate her priorities and her life. Clearly, her instinctual life had not been taken care of until now and seemed to be calling out to her urgently now that she was pregnant.

You can use this exercise for all sorts of dreams. Remember, you can rewrite the ending of a dream exactly as you wish or make up a new ending for a dream that feels incomplete. For instance, in a pursuit dream you might find out who you are running away from or what happens when you turn around and face your pursuer. In a house dream, you might find out what exists behind a closed door or discover a hidden room. Let your intuition guide you and this technique will lead you to all sorts of discoveries. Your dreams will never be the same again.

Painting and Drawing

There is a magic that happens when you translate a dream image from your unconscious mind onto a piece of paper or a canvas. Not only does it help you uncover new meanings for your dreams, it also enables you to identify hidden elements that have slipped past your rational mind. For example, in the above-mentioned dream about the puppy and the speeding driver, there was a group of witnesses surrounding the dog that were forgotten when the woman awoke from sleep. Only after she painted the dream did she discover who some of the witnesses were. She said that as she was painting, an image of a deer and a female angel appeared before her on the page. She had not expected this to happen. The mere act of painting conjured hidden dream elements into her conscious mind. The deer represented a particularly tender and vulnerable aspect, which she connected to the beginning of her pregnancy. The female angel seemed like a loving presence she had not expected to find inside her own psyche. She was an intensely self-critical person and this dream figure was definitely compassionate, even motherly. The dreamer associated it with the true nature of love and mothering. It reassured her to find it in her own dreams, as if this meant that she could become a good mother after all. She had been full of doubts and fears about the prospect of becoming a mother and not feeling equipped for it.

Painting is a very powerful exercise to use with your dreams because it does not involve the use of words. Painting allows you to transfer dream symbols directly to the outside world without any mental interference. It is for this reason that painting will often bring up aspects of your dreams that would otherwise stay locked in your memory banks. With painting, you are literally unmasking the unconscious, calling forth dream images that are heretofore unseen or forgotten.

As with the writing exercise, you can use painting to invent a new ending for your dream or change an ending that left you with a bad taste in your mouth. It is best before you lay your brush to the page to spend a few minutes in contemplation, going over the facts of your dream and fantasizing about new dimensions that your dreaming mind failed to express. Then, when you are ready, just let your brush or pencil begin its movement. As with the writing exercise, it is best not to censor yourself. If a wacky dream image wants to come out, just let it fly. The less you inhibit yourself, the better.

The great thing about this exercise is that even if you are not an expert painter, the very act of drawing or painting your dream images will awaken in you the skill necessary to complete the task. Something happens to our bodies when we attempt to speak or write our dreams. We become more alert, more awake, more conscious. Just paint your dreams and something miraculous will happen. Your artistic abilities will flare up. What was unseen before will enter your consciousness with clarity and ease. You will even remember your dreams better. The artist and the dreamer are connected. When you develop one, the other will follow.

EPILOGUE

"I am the cup bearer, come drink from me."

Science, philosophy, religion—all have delved into the mystery of life; each in its own way trying to contain, explain, understand what is in essence unfathomable, like the speed of light or the distances between two galaxies. I think poets have come the closest to grasping the indescribable beauty of life. From Rumi to Rilke and Yeats, they have thrilled us with the ecstasy of their soulful words. But never is that mystery more clearly embodied than in a woman pregnant with child.

Throughout centuries a woman's sexuality, her breasts, her vagina, her womb have been deified and reviled almost in the same breath, objectified so arduously that only the terrifying, awe-inspiring capacity to bring life forth can explain such a violent response to a woman's body.

This time of pregnancy is a sacred time in the life of a woman. It is an incomparable experience, like an idea, a song, or a poem waiting to burst forth and be heard. The dreaming life of a woman during pregnancy is always attempting to express aspects of this mystery. It gives us glimpses into the spiritual and emotional content of the pregnancy right through the labor itself.

Interestingly, for this book, all the women interviewed expressed the desire to have as natural a birth as possible, with the least amount of drugs that they could bear. They were also all ready and willing to breast-feed, knowing full well that nothing can replace this perfect gift of Nature.

One senses a trend among women today to reclaim their bodies from the medical machine and own the process of giving birth, however difficult or painful it might be. They are not afraid to look into the ancient mirror of creation and their dreams help them navigate through this ancient labyrinth like Ariadne's thread of gold.

The men and women interviewed in this book are the ones holding the thread outside the Minotaur's labyrinth. They are also the heroes venturing inside the cave and the ones emerging triumphantly because of the power of their intent to love in spite of doubts, worries, and fears about the awesome task at hand, the task of raising a child.

Through the dreaming life of these women who so honestly shared their stories with me, we have been able to look into this wondrous mirror of life creating itself moment by moment, like so many photographs.

Epilogue

I hope this book helps all of us, men, women, and future parents, to walk hand in hand through this journey of pregnancy with a little less trepidation and a little more trust in the wisdom of our own nature, recognizing all the while the heroic quality of all those involved, mother, father, and child.

To incarnate into a human being is an act of courage, and to take responsibility for such a creation to come through you is equally as worthy of praise.

For me, the process of writing this book was, in itself, a revelation and certainly an act of creation, which, like all such experiences, reveals more than one could ever "dream of"!

SUGGESTED READING

This reading list is by no means a complete list of books. It is simply a series of suggestions that cover as varied subjects as personal journeys into motherhood, the mystery and meaning of becoming a woman as well as a mother, the fine line between the scientific mind and the psychic mind, and of course comprehensive studies on the psychological nature of dreams.

Mother Mysteries by Maren Hansen (Shambhala Publications,1997). A fascinating and engrossing tale of a woman's three pregnancies as she comes to grips with the archetypal forces at work in the making of a mother. Human, holy, and earthy, a thoroughly spiritual experience as a book.

The Arsonist on Time by Raïna Paris (Raven Books, 1996). Poems and stories that tell of a woman's spiritual odyssey and historical perspective on the dreams and realities of her human destiny.

Inner Work by Robert A. Johnson (Harper San Francisco, 1989). A psychological perspective of dream interpretation by the best-selling author of *He* and *She*. Very helpful for using the realm of dreams as a tool for personal growth. A beautiful, fascinating book that is well written and a great psychological tool. I recommend it if you are serious about doing inner work from this perspective.

Having a Baby by Diana Bert, Katherine Dusay, Averil Haydock, Susan Keel, Mary Oei, Danielle Steel Traina, and Jan Yanehiro (Dell, 1985). A wonderfully entertaining and honest book written by seven pregnant women. Includes all the details of each of their pregnancies, from conception to giving birth. Informative, practical, real.

Second Sight by Judith Orloff, M.D. (Warner Books, 1995). This book opens the doors of perception between the rational and the psychic mind. It is the perfect bridge for all of the skeptics out there who do not trust their own psychic experiences and personal visions in their dreaming or waking lives. It also depicts the courageous journey of one woman to listen to the calling of her soul and integrates it in the medical arena.

Suggested Reading

The Woman's Encyclopedia of Myths and Secrets by Barbara Walker (Harper & Row, 1983). Truly a woman's bible. Filled with revelations about women's roles, Goddess mysteries, and everything you would want to know, from oracles to menstruating cycles.

GLOSSARY OF DREAM SYMBOLS

This glossary is by no means complete. It will give a general meaning to some of the symbols you have encountered throughout the book as well as a few others. You can also refer to the last two sections of the book for more detailed information about certain metaphors and settings. Once again, allow your own relationship to the dream symbol to pervade your response before you take in the meaning provided in the glossary. Let your own feeling response inform your evaluation of the metaphorical meaning of the dream image. Start your own glossary from your dream journal.

abroad: When you are pregnant, your own body can sometimes feel like a foreign country. The idea of becoming a mother can also be a strange and new concept, like being in a foreign country. Being abroad in a dream carries the symbolism of new growth and new experience. (Also check *travel* in Chapter Twenty, Part V, on themes.)

acorn: The seed that becomes an oak tree, a great metaphor for the process of pregnancy. This dream symbol could be reminding you to be patient, enjoy where you are right now, and stay with the process of what is being created here, rather than wishing it was over and the baby was here already.

acting: Could refer to a feeling that you are "playing the part" of the happy pregnant woman rather than really feeling it. Do you feel like a fraud? Inadequate? All these are common feelings for a first-time mother. You are better off bringing them to the surface and talking about them than not. They will have less power over you.

affair: This dream could be encouraging you to put more sex back into your life or simply reminding you that you are still a sexual being. You should probably ask yourself how you've felt about your sexuality since you have gotten pregnant.

animals: These types of dreams are always trying to tell us something about our instinctual nature. They are prominent during pregnancy, often trying to remind us to trust our instincts.

armor: Do you feel like you need protection, especially now that you are pregnant? What are you protecting yourself against? This could be a valid reaction to a current situation and how you view your pregnant state.

baby: Dreaming of a baby while you are pregnant or thinking about becoming pregnant is not unusual. You might want to pay attention to the mood of the baby, the setting, and how you are relating to the baby. This could give great insight into your own state of mind about becoming a mother, as well as the pregnancy itself.

baking: Another pertinent metaphor for pregnancy. If you are not pregnant yet, you might want to get a test. What are you baking? What stage of cooking is it at? Is your bun already in the oven or are you just getting started with the ingredients? What are your feelings in the dream?

bank: The dream could be telling you that you need to prepare for the upcoming arrival. It could be part of your nesting instincts. How are your finances? Are you storing things for the future? Do you feel secure or are you worried? Your attitude in the dream will let you know how you feel about this.

bath: Taking a bath is a reminder that you yourself can also feel like being in a womblike environment. Are you taking time to care for yourself? Do you feel like retreating from the world at this point of your pregnancy? These are all possibilities. Again, look at your attitude toward the bath you are taking in the dream. It will direct you to the right explanation.

bees: Bees are an ancient symbol. They make honey, a natural substance filled with healing properties. You might be feeling busy as a bee right now, getting ready for the baby. You could be the queen bee, producing all the nutrients to grow your baby strong and healthy. What is your reaction to the bees in the dream? Let it lead you to clarity.

birth: If you are close to term, dreaming of giving birth could be a premonitory dream or a rehearsal dream (Chapter Three, Part I). Trust your first reaction when you wake up from the dream as well as your feelings in the dream. Either way, the dream is usually helpful. It appears at the right time to prepare you for the big event. This can include exorcising your worst fears and conveying your fondest hopes.

candle: This could very well symbolize the new "light" growing inside you. It is a very spiritual symbol, both fragile and powerful at the same time.

cat: Cats are mysterious and sensual animals. Cat dreams could refer to your own sexuality, your instinctual life. Check with your own feelings in the dream. It could be a part of you that needs nurturing or special attention now that you are pregnant.

cathedral: See Chapter Nineteen on settings in Part V.

cave: See Chapter Nineteen on settings in Part V.

chocolate: Pregnant women often have food-related dreams. It could simply represent a craving or a need for sweetness in general. The dream could also be commenting on how sweet your life feels right now.

circle: A complete circle is a powerful symbol, an ancient mandala representing wholeness. This dream symbol could refer to how being pregnant makes you feel complete.

date: If you dream of a particular calendar date, this could very well be a premonitory dream for your labor. However, it could refer to other things as well. Are the numbers themselves meaningful to you?

The fruit is of course a different story altogether. A sweet and sensual fruit could refer to your connection to your sensuality right now. Some women actually feel very sensual when they are pregnant. Are you one of them?

dawn: A brand-new day is a perfect metaphor for the birth of a new child and a new mother. A very hopeful symbol.

deer: A beautiful gentle animal, which is also vulnerable. Do you feel like a deer caught in the headlights because you are becoming a mother? Are you scared, worried? Check with the feelings you had in the dream. This could also refer simply to your need for quiet and protection at this time.

doctor: Depending on your attitude in the dream, this could refer to your relationship to your doctor and how you feel about him or her. You might have some doubts or worries. Do not ignore them because it is "just a dream." You might also be needing to talk to someone, a spiritual doctor.

dolphin: An intelligent, powerful yet gentle animal, the dolphin has long been seen as a mythic animal and a friend to human beings. It is also an animal who is closely tied to the sexual feminine nature. Your attitude toward the dolphin, how connected you are to it in the dream, is paramount to your understanding of this symbol.

dress: If the dress is new, you might be tired of your pregnant look. If the color of the dress was important in the dream, how did it affect you? If you were "dressing up," maybe you need to make an effort in your waking life, even if you are "very pregnant."

dying: If you are the one dying in the dream this could very well mean that you feel as if a part of you is dying as you are accepting the fact that you will soon be a mother. Your dream is reflecting a transformation that is happening not only on a physiological level but also on a psychological one, both consciously and unconsciously.

ear: The shape of the ear is reminiscent of the fetus. So you could very well be dreaming about your future baby. As a matter of fact, in acupuncture, the whole body is represented in the ear alone.

earth: A desire to be connected to the earth could be at the "root" of this dream symbol. Refer to your attitude in the dream. If there is a sense of belonging to the earth, your pregnancy might be the cause. You feel part of the cycle of life in a way you have not before.

egg: This is an ancient symbol. The alchemists saw it as the "primordial" egg. This is a symbol that can appear at the onset of pregnancy, sometimes before you know you are pregnant. Pay attention to your attitude and to the color of the egg in the dream. Both can be revealing of your deep feelings about pregnancy and motherhood.

family: To dream of your family while you are pregnant could mean one of two things. Either you are feeling like you have a real family now that you are going to have a baby, or there are some things that you have not worked out with your family of origin and the unconscious feelings are in the way of your living joyfully this dream come true.

feathers: This dream symbol could be referring to the "heavenly" feeling that accompanies your pregnancy. It could be confirming your inner bliss. Or you feel like heaven has come down and blessed you with this baby you are now carrying.

fire: Depending on the type of fire, this dream symbol could be referring to several different things. If it is a small fire in a fireplace, it could mean that your pregnancy makes you feel warm and at home in your own body. If it is an intense fire in a big furnace but not threatening to you, it could refer to the creative process now taking place in your body. If it is an out-of-control fire somewhere, you could be feeling overwhelmed by the whole pregnancy thing and your hormones could be getting the better of you.

flowers: Flowers in bloom are beautiful, sweet-smelling, lovely things. You could be feeling this way, or the symbol could be referring directly to the pregnancy. In either case, you are feeling pretty good. However, if the flowers are in need of watering, it could be a direct plea from your body to drink more water.

forest: See Chapter Nineteen on settings in Part V.

fruit: This symbol is usually a reference to your attitude about life, whether you see it as rich, sensual, and abundant or not. It could also be a reference to the "fruit of your loins," the baby growing inside of you.

garden: A garden is almost always a metaphor for your inner life. When you are pregnant, it often symbolizes your relationship to your future baby and shows you your own growth as a result.

girl: This type of dream symbol could refer to your own childhood, a need to reconnect with her at this time of your life, a way to say good-bye maybe. It could also be a premonitory dream about the way your child will look at a certain age. Trust your feelings in the dream and your instincts about it.

gold: A magical element in many fairy tales and myths and the goal of the alchemical process, this substance is a powerful symbol. It could refer to your inner belief that becoming pregnant means that you have indeed "struck gold." The gold could also be a metaphor for the beauty and richness of the transformation taking place inside your body. Remember to look at the context in which this gold is set.

harvest: A harvest takes time to arrive. You plant things in the spring and harvest them in the fall. This dream could be telling you to be patient, that this pregnancy is part of the great cycles of Nature and your job is to be in tune with Mother Nature and accept its rhythm.

home: You may be in the process of moving into a new home; in such a case, you could be dreaming about your potential new home. Pay attention to your attitude toward the home in the dream; it could hold useful clues as to your true feelings about it. It could also be your general feeling of well-being at this point in your pregnancy.

honey: The rich sweet nourishing substance could be pointing you in a particular dietary direction. It could also be telling you that you need to treat yourself with love right now. It could also refer to the richness that your life is, preparing for the baby, being "busy as a bee."

husband: The context of the dream is essential here, how you relate to your husband, what you perceive he is doing and feeling, and so on. Are you wanting him to participate more in the pregnancy? Is he aloof or too busy with work? This could be useful information for your waking relationship.

infant: To dream of an infant is an obvious reference to the baby growing inside of you, but is there also a part of you that feels like "a brand-new baby"? In a sense you are a newborn mother, just as sure as your baby will be a "brand-new baby." Again, your attitude toward the infant in the dream could be a useful clue to your real feelings about becoming a mother.

infidelity: This dream might be telling you that you need to recognize that you are still a sensual and sexual being. Do you feel unattractive or is there a lack of sensuality between you and your husband right now? You might want to talk with him about it.

invisibility: Sometimes there is so much fuss made about your pregnant belly that you can begin to feel invisible. Perfect strangers feel free to come up to you and touch your pregnant body like it is a free-for-all. Check in with yourself about this. You might need to set some boundaries and ask your friends and family to talk about you as a human being as well as a baby maker.

island: A mother and her unborn child can feel like a special island far from everything and everyone. This dream symbol is a great metaphor for this state. Check with the dream and see how you feel about that. Is it a good feeling for you or does it make you feel isolated?

jewels: Precious jewels, like gold and pearls, are an ancient symbol for the inner self. For a pregnant woman, it also refers to the child she is carrying. There is no separation between the mother's soul, if you will, and that of her child at this point. He/she is the most precious part of her being. What kind of jewels are they? Do they have a special significance to you? Are they family jewels?

journey: The nine months of pregnancy are very much a journey for the mother-to-be as well as for the child she is carrying, so it is not unusual to have such a symbol in your dreams. What kind of journey is it? And how do you feel about it?

joy: To feel joy in a dream is a wonderful experience and pregnancy is certainly an occasion to feel joyous. How is this joy expressed in the dream? This dream could help you realize that despite some problems, this is actually a really happy time. Sometimes we foolishly hold back our joy. This dream is telling you to let it all hang out. Have the courage to be in your joy.

key: Depending on the context of the dream, this symbol could mean that you actually feel that you have found the "key" to a deeper happiness through your pregnancy. It could also refer to a sense of freedom you have not felt before. Of course, a key is also a very phallic symbol that could mean you are ready for a new level of sexuality in your life.

kitchen: There is something uncanny about the amount of metaphors that refer to cooking, baking, and so forth when it comes to creating a child. Most of these metaphors take place or relate in some way to the kitchen. This is the essential part of the house, a source of food and heat, which you are actually providing for your unborn child right now. Your attitude toward this kitchen in your dream is the key. Also pay attention to whether it feels natural or difficult in some way to handle the kitchen activities. This could refer to your reactions to pregnancy and motherhood.

knitting: This is an interesting symbol that could refer to the "web of your life." Do you feel that this pregnancy is an entanglement you did not really count on? It could also be referring to your desire to go back to old-fashioned values and nesting instincts that surface with pregnancy.

laboratory: This symbol is in many ways similar to the kitchen metaphor. Although this dream symbol is coming from a more "scientific" perspective, pregnancy still gives rise to this feeling that something is "cooking" in the womb. Something magical, even if it is being medically monitored, is happening. The point is the magic happening inside your body; *you* are creating this.

lake: Dreams of water abound during pregnancy. Perhaps you feel waterlogged physically. More than likely your pregnancy has taken you to a deeper realm, put you in touch with the unconscious mechanisms of your life, which are so prominently displayed right now.

lottery: You may be feeling as if you have won the lottery. Your pregnancy is an occasion to celebrate. It is a miraculous gift. You might also feel that you are taking a risk and that it is worth it. Again, check with your feelings about this in the dream.

mandala: This sacred circle is a symbol of wholeness. It is used in many Eastern religions as a focus for meditation. In a dream, it refers to your unconscious emphasis on this feeling, which is probably a result of your pregnancy. You might be reaching a sense of wholeness on a deeper level than you think.

massage: This could simply mean that you should treat yourself to a massage, a desire from the body making itself known through the dream. Massages are very relaxing and restorative; they help you to be in your body in a very loving way.

milk: This could be a premonitory dream about your breasts being ready to carry the milk necessary for your child. Or you could be feeling very motherly or like a cow ready for the milking. Whatever it is, check your attitude toward this symbol as it appears in the dream.

miscarriage: This is a typical anxiety dream for a pregnant woman, especially in her second trimester. Do not be alarmed, but listen to your intuition and by all means check with your doctor, especially if there is a history of miscarriage in your family. It is better to be safe than unnecessarily worried.

music: Maybe you just found out you were pregnant and it is "music to your ears." Or the pregnancy itself feels like you are listening to heavenly music or even creating it yourself.

nest: This could be a call to prepare for the upcoming arrival of your newborn baby. Are you someone who waits until the last minute to do something? Your unconscious might be telling you that it is time. Or the dream might be expressing the fact that your nesting instincts are in full swing at the moment. Check with your reactions in the dreams to find out where you stand.

nursery: Dreaming of such a symbol when you are pregnant makes perfect sense. It might be a very helpful dream if you have been undecided about the nursery's colors, look, and so on. Your soul could be trying to tell what the baby really wants. Pay attention and trust your intuition.

ocean: The most powerful symbol of the unconscious as well as the feminine nature of things. During pregnancy, you are the most in touch with this realm. It is also what happens in the "unseen" regions of life; it is where life began.

opening: Your pregnancy could be an opportunity for self-discovery, which opening a gift could be a symbol of. It could also be referring to the fact that the birth is imminent if you are attending an "opening" of some kind. If you feel a lot of excitement, that is also a very good clue that something important is happening or about to happen.

oven: A common metaphor for pregnancy, it could be letting you know that something is cooking if you have not had a pregnancy test yet. It could also simply be confirming that everything is cooking as it should be. Your feelings about this oven are essential for an accurate interpretation of the dream.

past: Dreams of the past are common at the onset of pregnancy (see Chapter One, Part I). Things come up in dreams because the unconscious is still holding onto them for whatever reason, happy memories or difficult ones. Your psyche thinks it is time to look at them and you would well be advised to take a look at what messages from the past are being offered for your perusal now.

path: Whether you are taking a stroll on a country lane or jogging through the forest can show you a lot about your reaction to your pregnancy and what kind of a journey it is for you. Is something familiar or strange? Is it pleasant or ominous? Your feelings in the dream will tell you what is really going on.

pregnancy: Dreams of pregnancy often come as a premonition, letting you know that you are actually pregnant. If the pregnancy is well under way, such dreams could also indicate how the pregnancy is going at this particular time.

queen: This could simply mean that being pregnant makes you feel like a queen, powerful, beautiful. It could also be warning you not to become a tyrant just because you are pregnant.

quilt: This could be an aspect of the nesting instincts revealing itself through this dream symbol of the quilt. It is also an old-fashioned familial art, something a mother or a grandmother would do. The dream could be showing you that you have some old-fashioned values inside of you longing to have a say at this time of your life. Again, how you feel about the quilt in your dream is paramount.

rainbow: Something beautiful is happening in your life, which is how you feel about your pregnancy, and the dream symbol of the rainbow is reflecting precisely that. Maybe you feel as if you got the "pot of gold" at the end of the rainbow. It might also be pointing to the fact that you need more colors in your life, your wardrobe, or your baby's room.

rest: Dreams are often a direct assessment of something you need in your life, so if this theme of "rest" appears in your dreamscape while you are pregnant you might pay attention to it. Are you doing too much for your condition? Is it time for you to cut back on activities so your body can devote all its energies to creating your baby right now? Or are you resting too much? These are just some of the questions you could ask yourself at this time. Consider your feelings in the dreams carefully.

room: New rooms in a dream usually refer to new parts of your psyche that were not available to you until now. Your pregnancy is an opportunity to look at "old rooms" from the past as well as "new rooms," including the room that is going to be the nursery. Pay attention to the type of room you are discovering, whether it is an old one or a new one, what is in the room, and if it is missing something. Of course, your own feelings are, as usual, an essential clue to the overall interpretation of the dream.

sanctuary: Sometimes with pregnancy comes a need for safety, protection, which such a dream symbol can represent. Either you are feeling that you have created a sanctuary in your life right now for you and your baby or that you still need to do so. What is the dream telling you?

seal: A seal, like the dolphin, is a mythical animal. It embodies the feminine instinctual and sexual energy. Your revelations will come from studying your relationship to the seal in the dream.

star: You could be feeling like the star of your own movie right now. If you are with a star in the dream, check what kind of qualities this star embodies for you. This dream could also be about a star in the night sky, showing you what a beautiful, bright being you are. (Check Chapter Three, Part I.)

time: If you are close to term in your pregnancy, this dream could be warning you that it is time to get ready for the big event, that you are running out of time for preparations, that now is the time.

traffic: In the third term of pregnancy, anxiety dreams often take on the common theme of things that can go wrong around the labor. In this particular case, you could be dreaming that you are caught in traffic on the way to the hospital and might have to give birth in the car. The dream might also be telling you that there is too much "traffic" going on in your life at this time and you might need to simplify things, to relax and focus on the upcoming event, the birth of your child.

twin: This dream could be about two entirely different things. Either you are dreaming of your own twin or if you do not have a twin, it means that you are dreaming of yourself as other or new. Maybe you are meeting the mother in you for the first time. On the other hand, you could be dreaming that you are going to have twins. In this case, you might be having a premonitory dream. You should definitely check with your doctor if it is not too early to detect what is going on.

underground: Psychologically and emotionally, your pregnancy may be pulling you "underground." You might just be in touch with the process happening in your body or your psyche might be telling you that now is the time for further exploration of your own depths.

uniform: Is motherhood some kind of uniform you dread putting on? Did you pick up your uniform from your mother or your grandmother? Your dream might help you figure out whether this is how you want to see motherhood, or maybe it is time to change your uniform, wear something new and different that is more like you. In any case, be sure to check how you feel about the uniform in the dream.

vegetables: Healthy, colorful, no-nonsense, these might be something to add to your diet when you are pregnant. Dreaming of vegetables might be a simple dietary suggestion from you to you.

victory: Victorious is what becoming pregnant may feel like to you. You are truly enjoying the fruits of your labor, carrying your child.

waiting: Patience when you are past your due date or even when you are in your third trimester is not necessarily a hallmark of pregnant women. This dream could be telling you, however, that at this point, you need patience and that it is a virtue. Of course, you can always talk to your baby and tell him/her to hurry up and come out. It has sometimes been known to work.

walking: When you are pregnant, your dreams often become full of information and suggestions about what you need to take care of yourself and your unborn baby. Walking might be one of those good ideas from your psyche. Of course, you might want to check how you feel about this walk in your dreams and if there is a particular destination.

weaving: An ancient craft, one of the domestic arts, a great metaphor for the process of creating a new life. What kind of weave are you creating? What colors? What textures? These are all clues for your pregnancy.

whale: If you are in your last trimester you might be feeling like a great whale. The whale is also a powerful symbol for the feminine creative energy of life and a clue as to how big of a deal this pregnancy really is. The size, color, and demeanor of this great mammal, as well as your reaction to it in the dream, are other clues for you to consider.

yard: If this is a backyard, it probably refers to your nesting instincts. You want your child to have a safe place to play. If this is a dream of the past in which you are the child playing in your family backyard or schoolyard, then you can be sure your psyche has some information for you to look at.

yoga: A great exercise for pregnant women. If it is coming up in your dream, you might consider adding it to your regime. Some classes are specifically tailored to pregnant women. If they are not available in your area, you might consider getting a videotape.

zodiac, the: A type of mandala, a sacred circle that could be pointing to the fact that you feel part of a whole, of the circle of life now that you are pregnant. Of course, if you are "into" astrology, it might have some other, more specific meaning.

zoo: Being pregnant, you sometimes feel like a caged animal, on display, under the scrutiny of too many solicitous family members. Dreaming that you are in a zoo could mean exactly that. It could be a warning before the pattern is too ingrained to set up some stronger boundaries and some alone time now.